BLOODY PRACTICE

BLOODY PRACTICE

DOCTORING IN THE CARIBOO &
AROUND THE WORLD

To Linda

STERLING HAYNES

Sterling Haynes

CAITLIN PRESS INC. 2003

Published by
Caitlin Press Inc.
Box 2387
Prince George BC V2N 2S6

Cover design and typesetting by Terra Firma Digital Arts.

Caitlin Press acknowledges the financial support from Canada Council for the Arts
and from British Columbia Arts Council for its publishing program.

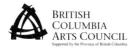
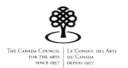

National Library of Canada Cataloguing in Publication Data

Haynes, Sterling
Bloody Practice: Doctoring in the Cariboo and Around the World

ISBN 0-920576-97-4
1. Haynes, Sterling. 2. Physicians–British Columbia–Cariboo Region–Biography.
3. Cariboo Region (B.C.)–Biography. I. Title
R464.H395A3 2003   610'.92   C2003-910477-X

CONTENTS

DEDICATION

This collection of short stories is dedicated to the women in my life. My wife Jessie and our four daughters; Elizabeth, Melissa, Jocelyn and Leslie. Jessie has been supportive and helpful, keeping me focused. Leslie has given me much constructive criticism, Elizabeth has been a tower of strength in helping me clarify my thoughts, in rewriting, organizing, and editing.

Circuitry of Laughter

The element of surprise
Sets off a circuitry of mirth.
A punch line or a pun
Stimulates guffaws, chuckles, giggles—
Contagious acts from the belly.

Emotions, ideas, sensations flow,
A tickle sparks
Brain's prefrontal cortex.
Currents of jubilation light the route
To a network of smiling facial muscles
That leave no choice
But to laugh along the way.

PART ONE

THE CARIBOO AND BEYOND

Frontier Practice

My first medical practice was in the Cariboo, at Williams Lake, British Columbia. This was the last frontier in 1960.

This wild country developed slowly from a tiny chapel, a Sepewecemic Indian settlement in 1840. The Cariboo Wagon Road to Barkerville's gold rush bypassed this hamlet in 1863. The "Lake" came into its own when the Pacific Great Eastern Railway arrived in 1919. The PGE RR has been known ever since as the "Please Go Easy" despite its modern name, BC Rail.

American and European ranchers settled the area. They ranched cattle and a few sheep and then with the clergy and politicians they ranched the Salish, Chilcotin and Carrier Indians. Everything was penned up nice and tidy with fences and reserves.

These were turbulent times with ranchers, loggers and miners trying to get their share of the wilderness. The Indians were trying to shake their yoke and the laws of alcoholic interdiction. There were battles royal on Saturday night in the Maple Leaf and Lakeshore Hotel bars.

I was the newest Doc and got my share of 'being on call' for most of the murders that occurred on the weekends as well as the massive trauma associated with mines, sawmills and logging. I was stationed in the doctor's room, which consisted of a toilet, a Lazy-boy chair and a telephone, by the front door of the hospital.

14   At that time the Cariboo Memorial Hospital was about fifty years old. It was a clapboard building, draughty, with a leaking roof above the emergency room. The outside gray paint was peeling and if, in winter, you left the front door open too long the furnace could blow out.

About a 100 feet way was a newer building—the chapel and morgue. This L-shaped building had two separate parts. The separation of the memorial altar from the post mortem metal table was by a greasy, bloody fingerprinted piece of canvas with draw strings that didn't work. The chapel was lit by candles and a 40-watt bulb, the morgue by two 40-watt bulbs. There was no heat, refrigeration or running water.

The building was constructed on the advice and money of an English woman, Countess Calonna de Montecchio in 1932—to honour her lover Lloyd "Cyclone" Smith, cowboy bartender, stampede arena manager and 'pick-up man'; and her brother Lieutenant E.C. Evans, RNR.

During the stampede in 1932 Cyclone attempted to pick up a cowboy on a bucking bronc. Cyclone's stirrup ripped off when the two horses collided. He fell and his head was crushed. He

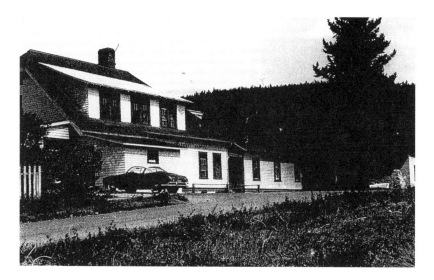

Williams Lake Memorial Hospital, circa 1958.
Photo courtesy of Irene Stangoe.

was placed in a wagon box and transferred to the concrete floor of a blacksmith's machine shop. The Countess was so incensed by the treatment of her lover that she built the morgue and chapel to honour her men.

To this day I can remember doing post mortems in dim light and seeing a bridle, a saddle with one stirrup missing and noticing the picture, naval uniform and sword belonging to Officer Evans on the opposite wall.

The hospital, office and morgue were where my professional life began. I became a country and urban physician, a real Doc.

Double Banged

3 am. Stampede Week in Williams Lake. I was drowsing in the Lazy-boy but wakened when the screen door banged. Joe went by me to the Emergency Room. He was unsteady. A trail of blood and sweat dripped down his face.

It was then I noticed the hatchet buried in his skull. It parted his long, black hair in the middle, the handle pointing forward. He was drunk. I jumped up and guided him to the Emergency Room stretcher.

"Don't lay down, Joe, for God's sake. Sit up and don't touch that hatchet."

Nurse Murphy was right behind me. "What happened to you, Joe?" she cried.

"Well, I was dancin' down at Squaw Hall, mindin' my own business, when my two friends double banged me."

"What the hell is double banged?" asked Murphy.

"You know, two against one. Two guys from the reserve jumped me and threw me onto the woodpile. There was this little hatchet for makin' kindling. They was going to scalp me with it but they didn't know how so they stuck it into my head and fell over laughing. I thought it was kind of funny, too, but then I started bleeding bad, Doc, and I walked up here."

"Who were these guys, Joe?" I asked.

"They're my buddies, Doc. I don't squeal."

"How could friends do this to you, Joe?"

"Friends just get like this!" said Joe.

"But this is serious. You'll have to stay in hospital while I figure how to get this out."

"No way, Doc. I can't miss the rest of Stampede. My brother Billy's bustin' broncs tomorrow. He could win."

"Just be patient, Joe. I'll have to call Vi in from X-ray to take some pictures to see where the hatchet is lodged and if it has cut your brain."

"I ain't got no brain, Doc. Just pull the sucker out."

I had visions of the blade embedded in the main sinus of the brain. If I wasn't careful, when I took it out there could be a massive hemorrhage.

I called Saddu, the lab tech, to come right away type and cross match for four pints of blood.

"Four pints of blood at 4 am, Dominion Day? We won't be able to find four donors at this time of night. Everyone is either partying or drunk. We only have about one hundred regular donors you know, Doc. I hope he's O-positive. I'll be right up. You'll have to phone the donors, though. I'm to scared to phone at this time of night."

Luckily, Joe was O-positive and was starting to sober up. After a number of phone calls, I found some sympathetic O-positive donors who agreed to come to the hospital and donate a pint of blood each. I hoped it would be enough. The x-rays showed the hatchet had split the skull and was probably lying in the sinus.

It was now about 7 am I phoned Jim Cluff, a Vancouver neurosurgeon, to explain the situation. Jim, in his precise way, told me exactly what to do.

"Be sure he's sober enough to understand and do it under local anesthetic," said Jim. "Phone back when you get things organized and I'll walk you through the procedure."

Murphy had started two IVs and we carefully moved Joe into the operating room. I got a phone extension to the operating room and called Jim.

"Take it easy," said Jim. "But do exactly what I say."

Slowly, I removed the hatchet. Luckily, there was a small hole in the superior sinus that was controlled with pressure. I laid gelfoam over the hole like a patch and held it with silk sutures.

"You're doing fine," Jim said. "Once you control the bleeding, the rest is a piece of cake. Phone me if you have further problems. I've got to run now." The telephone went dead.

Sweat ran over my glasses. It will be another hot, hot day at the Stampede I thought as I sutured the scalp wound.

"He didn't lose much blood," said Murphy. "Maybe a pint but we'll keep the IVs going."

Joe was moved to his ward bed and I went for breakfast.

When I came back, the ward nurse said, "Joe's never slept in a bed before and he wanted to sleep on the floor. I put the mattress under the springs. He's sound asleep now and his vital signs are stable."

I crouched beside him. The dressing was dry and he smelled of old whisky.

He did well over the next twenty-four hours.

"Have you got a headache?" I asked him.

"My head feels good, Doc, and I could eat a steak. I gotta see Billy win big tomorrow at the bronc riding."

"Joe, you've gotta stay here. You can't watch Billy ride tomorrow."

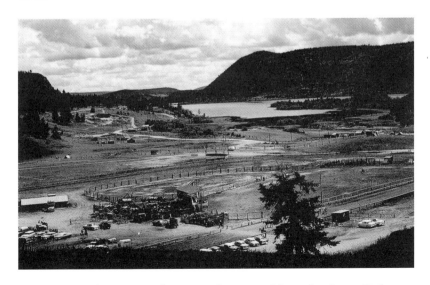

Williams Lake Stampede Grounds, 1958. Photo by Anna Roberts.

The next day, after lunch when the nurse picked up the tray, Joe was gone from under the bed. The cowboy in the next bed said, "Joe just had to watch Billy ride. Even after Billy and his cousin tried to scalp him! Billy brought him his clothes, boots and big Cowboy hat. They skipped out the back way."

An Emergency in the BC Wilderness

Thirty years ago, I had just started practicing in the small, frontier town of Williams Lake, in central British Columbia. I was fresh from a residency in California and still green, but keen and enthusiastic.

One Tuesday morning, a call came in: a light plane had crashed at One Eyed Lake in the Chilcotin, an area of jack pine, swamp, stump ranches and Indian reservations about 130 miles west of Williams Lake on a plateau between the Rocky Mountains and the Coast Range.

Being the junior man of the four practitioners, I was "elected" to go on the mercy flight. I had been on call all week. It was supposed to be my day off.

I phoned my wife from the hospital to tell her I'd be gone again and collected the equipment I'd need: emergency room bag, a frame wire stretcher, bottles of dextrin and saline, needles and Thomas splints. I had trouble loading everything in my VW. Beetle. The stretcher ended up partly in the back seat and partly out of the window. Off I went in a cloud of dust (there being few paved roads in Williams Lake at the time) to find my pilot, Colonel Joe.

Colonel Joe was an American, a Southern gentleman who had flown with the Flying Tigers under General Chenault in Southeast Asia. He was now working as a bush pilot, flying his Cessna 180 in the rugged central BC wilderness.

I finally found him at the float plan wharf on the east side of Williams Lake, using a hand pump to fill his plane with gas from a forty-five gallon barrel.

We started loading the equipment but couldn't figure out what to do with the stretcher. Then we hit on it: we'd lash it horizontally across the front of the pontoons. We threw the bags, dextrin and splints into the plane. I closed the passenger side door and Colonel Joe pushed off and paddled out onto Williams Lake. The prop eventually caught and we taxied down the lake. As we turned into the wind, I wondered if this "white knuckle" airline would get me to my destination and back again with the patients. Colonel Joe had only a vague idea where One Eyed Lake was and I had none.

We took off and flew lazy circles around the lake to gain altitude for the journey west. We passed over the Fraser River at about 1500 feet and followed the road up the Sheep Creek Hill. At the top of the hill, the Chilcotin lay unveiled before us covered in smoke. A massive forest fire was blazing. The smoke obscured the roads, the lakes were only hazy blotches beneath us. Flames hot up about three hundred feet, the sparks shooting even higher. The heat was so intense and the smoke so dense that we had to climb higher.

After circling for what seemed like hours in that droning machine, we spotted Puntzi Lake and the US Puntzi Mountain Early Warning System airstrip. At Colonel Joe's request, I fumbled around the tail of the plane looking for a topographic map. I found the one we wanted. The map section with One Eyed Lake was missing. Colonel Joe was non-plussed.

"We'll look for the lake all day if we have to," he said. "Or until we run out of gas."

The smoke was starting to disperse in the west and Colonel Joe dropped lower until we were skimming the tree tops trying to figure which of the many lakes in the area might be One Eyed. Suddenly we saw a lodge and a man waving. Then we heard two shots from his side by side shotgun. This was the lake.

We circled the area looking for log snags and a safe place to land. "Don't want to put a hole in one of the goddamned pontoons," said Colonel Joe. "Then we'd be in a hell of a fix. You can swim, can't you, Doc?"

The landing was smooth and Cappy, a retired British officer, met us at the wharf. We unloaded the equipment with the help of two young Chilcotin Indians.

The downed plane was in a field about a quarter of a mile away. The pilot was dead. The man in the seat beside him was alive, but barely. A young boy, sitting among some sleeping bags in the back, had only injured his ankle. The sergeant medic and a corporal from the US base at Puntzi were at the site, trying to pry open the passenger door of the plane to get the injured man out. The prop and engine had been driven into the mud, making the door extremely difficult to budge.

We managed to pry it open and slowly lifted the injured man onto the wire stretcher. His curled up position and seat belt had saved him. He was semi-conscious and in shock from multiple fractures. His scalp had been torn off. I looked around, found it by his seat and wrapped it in a lunch bag. I cleaned his mouth with my fingers, removed bits of broken teeth with gauze and inserted an oral airway. I searched for a large vein without a fracture around it and started dextrin. We splinted the fractures as best we could. With dextrin running in each arm and the two young Indians carrying the bottles, the four of us started through the woods for the plane.

The patient began to scream. We stopped and I gave him two milligrams of IV morphine. A bad mistake. Within a minute he had stopped breathing. Shock and morphine had totally depressed all respiration. I had to intubate him in a mud hole with flexible rubber endo-tracheal tubes and only a small portable oxygen tank. After twenty minutes we started moving again and the patient started screaming, thank God.

Back at the lodge, we sent the two medics back to get the boy with the injured ankle. Colonel Joe proposed we strap the stretcher to the pontoons, covering the man with a canvas tarp to prevent him from getting too wet. I vetoed that idea. It was

Cappy who suggested we use his radio to contact the RCMP detachment at Williams Lake to see if they would fly in with a larger plane.

After much static and crackling, Cappy managed to get through and they agreed to fly the Beaver down from Prince George. Colonel Joe decided to fly back and notify the hospital that we'd follow with the two patients.

By the time the plane arrived at noon, the normal saline and dextrin were almost used up. The patient's vital signs were present but his blood pressure was 80/?. We moved the seats to accommodate the basket stretcher and with IV bottles strung from light switches, we reached Williams Lake. The plane taxied to Colonel Joe's wharf where we were met by the mortician who doubled as an ambulance driver and the hearse which doubled as an ambulance. We loaded the patient into the hearse and were off in a cloud of dust.

I stayed with the patient for 24 hours. We pumped blood, sewed lacerations, re-sutured his scalp and applied plaster splints. Thirty-six hours later, the Air/Sea Rescue arrived from Vancouver to transport him to the Vancouver General Hospital where he was to stay for the greater part of the next three years.

Thirty years later, I'm on a locum in Nakusp, a south-eastern town in BC about three hours from anywhere. Another emergency, this time a man with acute myocardial infarction. We transfer him by air to Kelowna. Monitors, life packs, nitroglycerin, a lidocaine drip and IV morphine are set out in a well-equipped ambulance which rushes us to an airstrip on the outskirts of town. A small jet with state-of-the-art stretcher and equipment are waiting there.

We're off in a matter of minutes, and minutes later we're in the ICU of Kelowna General Hospital. The cardiologist is waiting. The patient is dozing and comfortable.

Chummy

The gravel roads and sidewalks in Williams Lake, B.C. are icy. The Medical Clinic lights go off and the street darkens. I carefully step into the street.

"Bloody raw, could be getting colder, Doc" said a voice.

"Is that you Chummy? Ah—now I see you. Better button up that old army battledress. That khaki looks threadbare."

"Yeah Doc, that chill can get you. Need whisky for the frost on my bone. The dogs yapping and the coyotes howling make it seem colder," said Chummy.

The Doc knew that Chummy had been drinking since the Christmas party at the Legion. Shrapnel wounds and alcohol were making him sick.

"Yeah, since D-day the remittance cheques from my family have been slow in coming. Since haying time in the Chilcotin that rancher Ten Percent Joe hasn't paid me a red cent."

Chummy had been a sergeant once, a leader of men. He'd been mentioned in dispatches and won the military medal. He could sing Handel's Messiah, had a sweet tenor voice. Sometimes he would recite the poetry of Burns and Tennyson in the bar.

I can remember his rendition of Ulysses even now:

"Though much is taken, much abides, and though we are not that strength, which the old days moved heaven and earth, that which we are we are."[1]

"I hope you don't mind me saying so but you better do up your fly Chummy, may be detrimental to your privates."

"Please not again, Chummy."

"I need "Oh hell, not to worry —Sir Winnie always said, 'a dead bird never leaves the nest.' I'm feeling despondent since Mary and the kids left. I think I'll tie one on again tonight."

"I need a drink. I'm Chummy, a Canadian now. No more James Chomondely the Third."

I shook hands with Chummy and watched him stagger down toward the Ranch Hotel bar. That was the last time I was to see him alive. Perhaps the rest of his evening went something like this:

A door slammed and the sound of Western music from a Wurlitzer fills the bar: "I found my thrill on Blueberry hill."

"Hi Chummy, have a beer with the old gang," cried his buddy Mac. "Have a drink and tell us about the Italian campaign, Christmas 1943, wasn't it?"

In that campaign it was mostly the Loyal Edmonton Regiment and the Seaforth Highlanders against the German Panzer division. They were tough. The Canucks were under General Vokes.

Yes," said Chummy."It was mayhem in ice and mud. I was struggling with my platoon coming up from the south. Ortona, on the Adriatic, was held by the Panzer division. The Krauts were dug in around a high promontory flanked by sea cliffs and a deep ravine. The Germans had an armored division. We had the 'Hallies', the Halifax bombers from the number 6 RCAF bomber command and some artillery. We blasted the Krauts for days. On December 20, 1943, Vokesy ordered the infantry in."

"Was it brutal?"

"Yeah, some of my buddies died at first but we made it through and captured a hill close to the main promontory. From there on it was hand to hand combat. On December 27th, we took Ortona, the same damn day I was wounded. We fought in the streets. I was up to my ass in shit. Tracers flashed everywhere, machine gun bullets ricocheted off the marble walls. We ran, hid, then ran, shooting our Stens. We took German pill-boxes with grenades and flame throwers. I can still hear them shriek and sizzle now as we fried those Germans. The artillery on both sides started up, shrapnel burst in air and off buildings. It was chaotic, men fell, screaming and groaning 'til the stretcher bearers found them. They did what they could, gave them morphine and set up IV's of plasma, bound their wounds and bundled them off to the rear. I can see the medics now—faces covered with sweat, their battle dresses steaming from exertion as they carried the stretchers out of the line of fire."

"Was that the day you were awarded the military medal and wounded?"

"Yeah, my the wounds were superficial and the men gathered their strength and we broke through the German Gothic line and went on to Rimi. That was a blood bath in mud. Many of my buddies from the Cariboo died."

Cannon to right of them
Cannon to left of them
Cannon behind them
and thundered
They that had fought so well
Come through the jaws of death,
Back from the mouth of hell
 All that was left of them,
Left of six hundred." 2

"Geeze, was it that bad? Have another pint on me Chummy," said Mac.

"Let's drink for those dead blokes. Maybe I can forget it all and Mary too."

"Hey waiter, another round of beer," shouted Mac.

 The Wurlitzer song started again: "I found my thrill on Blueberry hill."

I wasn't there to see Chummy come out of the bar, but heard it was like this:

Six hours later the bar door slammed and a bleeding

Chummy crashed into the street. His breath a frozen cloud, battle dress undone, belt askew, galoshes flapping and pants open as he fell into the snow.

"I don't want to see you again until you sober up and get some money," said the bouncer.

"Yes sir, Captain, expect I'll wander back to my shack in Smedleyville."

"That's four miles."

"Hell I'm tough, I'll make it."

"Be careful. I can hear them huskies howling," said the bouncer. "They dragged a moose down on Second Avenue last Sunday night."

"No bother, I'm on my way. I'll quick step it home."

The moon came out and reflected the glassy black surface of the frozen road.

Dripping blood from his nose and a gash on his right hand, Chummy half-marched and half-slipped down the road. He heard the coyotes howling and he could see the sleigh dogs fighting among themselves in the distance. As he got closer, he saw that the pack had one of their own down and in a blood lust were tearing the animal to pieces. A few yips and it was all over.

"Jesus," he whispered, turning and running back to the street lights at the edge town. The pack gave chase. Chummy picked up a tree limb in the ditch and ran for a big Douglas fir.

Yipping, they came for him, their bellies close to the ground, slavering, snarling. He ran to the tree, swung his club at the first one, a gray shadow. The dog yipped as the limb broke in two. A second dog leapt for his left leg, Chummy felt a searing pain and a rip. "My God, I'm hamstrung," he thought as he lashed out with the broken club. His hands were too slippery with blood and the weapon slid from his hands. He tried to make it to the fir tree but a second dog slashed at his throat, the pack closed in.

"Someone help me," cried Chummy. The pack dragged him into the ditch.

A police cruiser's headlights picked up the pack of snarling dogs in the ditch and blood in the snow.

"A pack of dogs have somebody in the ditch," bellowed the constable into the his radio. His spotlight picked up the shine of a galoshes' buckle. "I'll need backup now."

Three shots rang out, three dogs went down, the other six ran.

"Its Chummy. He's badly mauled, get the ambulance, call the Doc"—the policeman shouted into his radio.

Mary and the three kids and townspeople gathered at the cemetery, on a cold winter day to bury Chummy. At the bar the patrons all chipped in to pay for the gravestone. Doc read the eulogy, the closing words taken from Burns.

"For a' that and a' that,
It's coming yet, for a' that,
That man to man the world o'er
Shall brothers be for a' that" [3]

On the icy granite marker was chiseled:

James Alexander Chomondely 111
1918 – 1959 M.M.
"That which we are, we are —
one equal temper of heroic hearts"
from Ulysses CHUMMY
by Tennyson

1 Tennyson, Alfred Lord, "Ulysses."
2 Tennyson, Alfred Lord, "The Charge of the Light Brigade."
3 Burns, Robert, "For A' That and A' That."

(This story is a work of fiction but was inspired by a similar death of a World War Two veteran on the streets of Williams Lake, in 1960)

Meningitis in the Chilcotin

The white glare of the policeman's flashlight shone in my eyes as I struggled up from sleep.

"What the hell is going on?" I asked, reaching for the bed lamp.

"Sorry, Doc," said the giant cop dripping melting snow all over the carpet. "You knocked the phone off the hook and Muriel at the hospital wants you right away. Sister Robert just arrived from the Alexis Creek reservation with six sick babies. They look pretty bad to me, Doc. Sister said the roads were awful, she slid all the way down Sheep Creek Hill."

"O.K., Constable. I'll be right over. Don't wake my wife and kids on the way out."

"Drive careful, Doc, it's snowing and slippery as hell."

I dressed hurriedly, slung on my Macinaw and buckled my overshoes, tiptoeing out of the house so as not to wake our new baby. The carport was snowed in. My breath frosted the cold dawn and my mustache grew icicles as I shoveled.

Snow crunched under the Ford's tires as, gripping the steering wheel, I slipped sideways down the hill. The chains rattled against the chassis and fenders. Finally, the lights of the War Memorial Hospital wheeled into view. Somebody has shoveled out the front entrance, but the heavy snowfall was filling in the valleys. Everything was white.

My footprints were the first to pass Sister Robert's battered van, covered with snow and frozen slush. She must have been desperate to drive those roads and send the Constable to root me out.

A warm blast of air fogged my glasses, as I opened the hospital door. "He's coming now," I heard Sister Robert tell the matron, Iris. "His mustache is covered in ice."

The sister's face was drawn, her white wimple accentuating her tanned, lined face. Her grey habit echoed the soberness of the situation. Light from the forty watt bulb of the emergency room glistened off her gold cross.

"How was your trip in, Sister?"

"Bad. Veasey is behind me with his truck and camper. He's got studded tires and makes slow progress. This time of year you have to have chains. Another seven babies are with his mother in the camper. They're all under a year, and I only brought the sickest of the thirteen. I thought it was pneumonia when I first saw them, but they all got sick at once and some had running ears. Do you think it could be meningitis, Doc?" she asked, fingering her rosary.

"Could be. Can you stay to help? We have a real emergency on our hands if it's meningitis."

"Sure, I'd rather drive back after the snowplow has been through, anyway."

"We'll need more cribs and bassinets. There are some stored in the Memorial Chapel and Morgue. The mattresses may be frozen. Let me take a look at the kids."

I peered into one of the cribs. "This little guy is Ray Johnny. He's about ten months old. I almost lost his mom on the x-ray table so she named him Ray."

Ray was quiet, the fontanelle bulging, his neck stiff and his eardrums red.

"You're a good diagnostician, Sister—it looks like meningitis. We'll need to do lumbar punctures on all of them. I'll call Donald to come and help, the other two doctors are away."

"And not coming back anytime soon. The airport is closed, nothing flying in or out," said Muriel. "If it's meningitis, the kids will have to stay here. I'll get all the available nurses and aides in.

We can use you for as long as you can stay, Sister."

"Sure. I've nursed babies with meningitis before."

It was a long, grey dawn. The snow piled up, drifting across the silent town, obliterating the trees and lake.

The door blew open, Veasey and the seven babies and Donald rushed in.

"My God!" Donald's Scottish brogue echoed down the hospital corridors. "I didn't see kids as sick as this in Edinburgh, never saw snow like this in Edinburgh. Wish to hell I was still in Edinburgh."

"We'll manage, Donald, once we get all the cut downs running. We may have to stay here alternate nights."

"I'm game," said Donald. "We don't have a choice, the blizzard could last a week."

So began the long vigil, with Sister Robert in charge of the babies, cut-downs, IVs and multiple antibiotics.

After ten days, the babies were much better. The roads were cleared and a January thaw was starting. The announcer at the Williams Lake radio station issued twice daily bulletins for the parents to come and get their children:

"Jimmy Johnny in Nemiah Valley, come and pick up your son. Johnny at Tasiniah Lake Lodge, tell Mac Quilt to leave the fencing job and drive in to get Emily." Sister Robert would get on the radio to ask for parents to pick up their kids at the hospital. She took some of them home in her battered van.

I ran into Sister in the hospital before she returned to the reserve.

"Thanks, Sister, your help has been invaluable. Those cut downs were the life lines and without IV Fluids, antibiotics, and your nursing care, all those babies would have died. Your astuteness in assessing them babies initially saved their lives. Why did you join the order, anyway, sister?"

"I wanted to help spiritually and practically as a Grey Nun. I've done it for twenty years, Doc. I work best in lonesome places like the Chilcotin. I love the people. They trust and depend on me."

34   Sister Robert was recalled to Montreal for a two year religious retreat. Rumour had it that her superiors felt she'd lost touch with God.

Thirty-seven years later, I went to the new Cariboo Memorial Hospital to look at the records of those thirteen babies. The charts had disappeared. And Sister Roberts never returned to the Chilcotin.

Shooting at Horsefly

"I just shot Lou through the guts with a 30-30 and drug him into the Horsefly River."

4 am, Halloween day. I pulled myself up in bed. "Hold on, Ingrid. Is he dead? Where are you phoning from?"

"He's dead now and I think he was dead when I drugged him into the river. I'm phoning from Lou's ranch house."

I knew both Lou and Ingrid. Lou was a sick old rancher who lived close to Horsefly Landing on a small stump ranch. He ran a few cows of mixed breed. Ingrid was a German immigrant in her early twenties. She'd come to Canada as a teenager and worked for Lou as his housekeeper. Lou was cantankerous. Suffering from angina and heart failure, he was morose and depressed usually.

Ingrid was paranoid most of the time. Three months before, she'd shaved off all her body hair, including eyelashes, to prevent evil thoughts and voices from entering her. When asked about it, she said "It's my body, isn't it?"

As soon as I gathered my wits, I shouted into the phone. "Put the gun away. Stay in the ranch house, and I'll be out with the constable as soon as I can. Do you understand, Ingrid?"

Ingrid said she understood.

I phoned the Williams Lake RCMP office and told the night constable what has happened. I said I'd be up to the police station right away. I told him we'd need a stretcher, hip waders and grappling hooks.

We roared out to Horsefly, about thirty miles away, sliding around the many turns in the gravel road. It was the cold hour before dawn when we drove into the yard. The house was ablaze with light. Ingrid had made coffee. We found her in front of the mirror, plucking out her eyelashes and talking to herself.

"Ingrid, where's Lou now," I asked, as calmly as I could.

Ingrid looked at me as she continued to pluck. Finally, she said, "as soon as I get these bad hairs out and the bad voices stopped, I'll show you. What's your hurry, Doc? He's dead and isn't going anywhere."

At dawn, Ingrid put down her tweezers and said, "Come on, I'll show you where I rolled him into the river after I roped him and pulled him with my horse. I shot him about four feet from where you're standing, Doc. He made a bloody mess of the floor."

She took us down to the river. By the early light, we spotted Lou's body hooked on a snag in the icy waters. The constable put his hip waders on and waded into the fast flowing water with the hooks. After several tries, he managed to catch Lou's long underwear and between the two of us, we pulled him ashore. The water was frigid. Lou was stone cold dead.

We called the mortician at the Lake. The "Goose," as he was known to his friends, agreed to come for the body with his hearse/ambulance. When he arrived, we loaded frozen, stiff Lou into the hearse. Then the constable, Ingrid and I rode in the police cruiser back to town.

In town, I notified the coroner. We took Ingrid to the hospital. Sitting on the stretcher in the Emergency room, she plucked hairs from her arms. "Those goddamned hairs are giving me bad nerves, Doc, and the voices are telling me to do mean, mean things."

I got my colleague, Hughie, to help me fill in the "pink form" to allow us to send Ingrid to the provincial mental hospital at Essondale. We got a constable and police matron to take her there. I thought I was finished after Ingrid left, but then the coroner phoned me to do the autopsy that night.

Lou's body had been deposited in Memorial Chapel and Morgue behind the hospital. The morgue was at the back of the chapel, behind a curtain. There was no heat, no running water. The place was lit by two forty watt bulbs. Lou, still in his long underwear, was on the sloping, drained metal slab with a block of wood under his head.

It was in this austere building that I performed my first autopsy in Williams Lake. Lou had been shot at close range with a 30-30. The entrance wound, mid-abdomen, was covered with powder marks. The exit wound was gaping. Part of his lumbar vertebra and aorta had been taken out. His left coronary artery was arteriosclerotic in the anterior descending portion and his lungs were wet from chronic passive congestion. Death was due to the bullet and was instantaneous although Lou could have died at any time from heart disease.

It was 9 pm when I left the morgue. The rickety wooden sidewalk was enshrouded by moonlight. A typical Halloween night marked by the lonesome cries of the last few ghosts and goblins yelling "trick or treat."

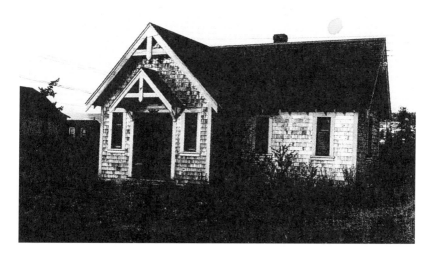

Chapel and Morgue, circa 1958. Photo courtesy of Irene Stangoe

Nechi – My Spirit Touches Yours

It was midnight and the phone rang again. Was this a long night starting on call?

"Hello, doctor, this is Nurse Murphy in Emerg. Ruby is here again from Alkali Lake. She's been beaten, her face is a mess and her right hand is painful. Vi is coming to take x-rays. She says you delivered her son here at the Cariboo Memorial hospital a year ago."

"Thanks, Murph. I'll be down in about 20 minutes. Better get Vi to x-ray her facial bones, nose, right hand and anywhere it hurts."

It was a winter night after Christmas, frigid and crisp. The Chevy's tires crunched snow into the road.

Entering the hospital, I wondered what her injuries were this time.

"Hi, Ruby. Ouch, you look sore. How are you feeling? How's your family?" I asked.

Ruby was sitting in a white hospital gown on an emergency room stretcher. Her face was puffy and purple, her eyes almost swollen shut, her nose displaced to the right. Her right hand was cradled in her left.

"Yeah, I'm hurting. The kids is good, Doc, but I ain't married now. I got into an argument five days ago and I lost! I'm late cause the stage ain't running, got no more money and I had to wait for a ride. I stopped drinking last year, I'm teetotal now. My kids won't stay with me if I drink. Iris, the oldest, forced me into it. She's hard-headed, you know," Ruby said.

"But who beat you?"

"Well, Doc, I won't say but I gave him a good right-hand punch before he got me down and put the boots to me. I can only eat slop but I'll manage."

"If you know who beat you up, Ruby, we can lay charges with the police," I urged.

"I can't talk, Doc. Our people are handling the problems our way now. The priest is no help. I don't go to confession anymore. Besides, Doc, we don't want some young, white cop messing around our reserve. No more Alcohol Lake, most of friends have sworn off the booze. It's Alkali Lake again, Doc."

I was glad to hear it. Alcohol had been a big problem with the Salish and Metis peoples on the reserve for years.

"Well, that's great, Ruby. What did you say about the priest?"

"The priest has been drunk since New Year's Eve and he's not concerned about us. The kids are going to school and we run the bootleggers off. If we can stop the Dog Creek stage from bringing the whiskey and beer, things will get even better. Sometimes the bus is so full of home brew and drugs, there's no room for passengers," Ruby proclaimed.

"How is the Band doing?" I asked.

"Doc, my friend, we're using our own spirits not the white man's. We're getting our old ways back, respecting the elders. We're remembering our earth mother, the pow-wow, the sweat lodge and sage burning. I know how our people live, I see how they die! We need our learning, trusting, remembering to help with healing. We need to speak our own language. No white cops. Just fix my nose, doc."

"Have you eaten recently?"

"Hell no, he knocked a bunch of teeth out."

I examined Ruby then looked at the x-rays on the view box.

"Well, Ruby, you've got a badly fractured nose. We'll have to reduce the fracture. You have a boxer's fracture below your right little finger which should heal fine in a splint. You'll have to see a dentist tomorrow. I just wish I knew who did this to you."

"You just don't get it, Doc, do you? Our people lost their mar- bles, but we're getting them back now. One marble for each month we're teetotal. We give them out in the sweat lodge," she said with a lopsided grin.

"You sure you don't want to tell?"

"I know you and trust you, Doc. Now you gotta trust us. We're trying to change in our own way. Just fix the nose, Doc. You might say I broke it putting it into other people's business."

An Unkindness of Ravens

Jim tottered through the doorway of the emergency room of the Cariboo Memorial Hospital at 3 am. He smelled of rum, but that wasn't unusual for Stampede Week in William Lake in 1960.

"Sorry to bother you, Doc," he said. "You know since I won that million in the Irish sweepstakes I been partying lots. But lately, I been feeling kinda sick, kinda smothery, like my tank's on empty. You know what I'm saying, Doc?"

I helped him onto the examining table.

"Have you been taking your medicine, Jim?"

"Well I forget sometimes. You know, Doc, my legs gets so swollen sometimes I can't get new Tony Lama boots on. Them boots is snakeskin and now I have to wear these moccasins."

I looked Jim over. He was dressed in stampede garb—stovepipe jeans and a western pearl button shirt. He was a mid-sized guy from the Sugarcane Reserve with raven black hair and an oriental cast to his black eyes. He was in bad shape. His nose, lips and nail beds were blue. His neck veins were distended, his chest rattled and his legs were swollen to his knees. I admitted him to the hospital and started oxygen, thiomerin and digitoxin. He seemed to improve. I arranged for him to be seen in a week by a cardiologist at St. Paul's Hospital in Vancouver.

A few weeks later the screen door of the hospital banged. I looked up and there was Jim and Wolfgang. Wolfgang was the

44   owner of the Williams Lake Chrysler dealership. Jim was dripping wet and covered in mud.

"Gee, Jim, you're a mess," said Nurse Murphy. "Been for a
morning swim?"

Jim grinned sheepishly. "Sort of."

"Did you see the heart specialist?" I asked as Jim climbed out
of his muddy pants.

"Yeah, I went down there just like you said. I bought me a
brand new Cadillac after I seen the Doc there. Then me and my
buddies headed straight home. Well, we stopped for a few beers
at Hope. At Boston Bar, Lytton, Ashcroft, Clinton, and 100 Mile
House, too. Damned if one of them tricky curves around the
lake didn't get me and we ended up in the drink."

"How'd you get home, Jim?"

"We hitched. The boys wanted to stop at the Chilcotin Inn,
but I needed to get a new car."

"Doc, he came waltzing into the dealership like this. Wanted
to buy a new Chrysler, you know the yellow one I got in the
showroom. He threw me the keys for the Cadillac, which he said
was stuck in the lake mud just out of town. Said I could have it.
He didn't look good so I brought him here."

"Thanks, Wolfgang," I said. "So, Jim what did the specialist
say?"

"Says I need a new valve job, Doc. Kinda like my car, haha.
Supposed to go down again at roundup time in the fall. She told
me just what you said, Doc. 'Take your medicine, lay off booze,
smokes and peanuts.'"

"You better go down for that heart operation," I told him. I
knew he'd die without it.

"Christ, Doc. I got money to spend before they cut me. I better get started."

I advised Jim to take his medicine, stop the booze, and check
with me every week.

But I didn't see him until Labour Day. I'd heard he'd been
busy smoking and drinking, telling stories and eating salted
peanuts. I asked Sister Robert, at the RC Mission on the reserve,

to talk to him. She had but to no avail.

I decided I'd have to track Jim down. If his buddies knew about his condition, maybe they'd help. So late one September evening I ventured into the Ranch Hotel bar. It was packed and smelled of stale beer, urine and smoke. Country music blasted from the jukebox in the corner. I found Joe at a table surrounded by his raven-haired buddies. Some were dancing around the table.

"Hey, Doc, take a load off," said Jim.

"Thanks Jim, but I can't stay. You haven't been in to see me or get your shots. I hope you're taking your pills."

A couple of guys danced past.

"Jim, could you ask your friends to stop their prairie chicken dance and listen. I'd like to talk to them."

"Doc, you got us mixed up with those Blackfoot out on the prairies. I could ask them to stop but I doubt they'd talk to you, Doc."

"Well, how are you feeling?"

"Not too good – I cough all the time and now blood is coming. The boys say its TB, nothing wrong with my heart. It's too noisy to talk here and they's having too much fun."

With that Jim stood up, ordered drinks for the house, then collapsed back into his chair.

In October, I received a call from the cardiologist in Vancouver saying Jim had missed his appointment and surgical booking time.

Nurse Murphy called me at midnight on Thanksgiving. The ambulance had just brought Jim in from the Riske Creek Rodeo where he'd collapsed. When I got to the hospital Jim was short of breath, blue, and his legs were swollen.

"Jim, why didn't you come and see me before, like I said."

"We was having too much fun," Jim replied between deep gulps of oxygen. "I couldn't miss spending the money. It's been six months since I won. Still got a few hundred bucks left, Doc—tucked in the toes of my Tony Lamas. Some say that Irish money is killing me, Doc. What do you think?"

I paused started the IV and the resuscitation but Jim continued to deteriorate. He died three hours later. He was thirty-
seven years old.

Johnny Mack

"Hi Mrs. Mack, has Johnny gotten worse?" I ask as I stride into the emergency room of the Inland Memorial Hospital.

"Yes, much worse."

"Why didn't you bring him in before now?"

"Since your nurse Margaret was so rude to me, we have decided to switch doctors. We see Dr. Jim now. That's why we're here in the hospital with Johnny."

"I didn't see you for a follow up and there was no answer on your home phone. Is that Johnny's cough I hear?"

"Yes, he started in again with fever and rapid breathing. His croup has gotten worse. He's in a croup tent with oxygen. But Dr. Jim's in charge."

"Apparently, he can't be found," I muttered under my breath.

"Now you look here, Doctor," said Mr. Mack as he joined his wife. "Don't give us any hassle."

"Johnny's only two you know—he's my dear sweet boy," added Mrs. Mack.

Johnny was a handsome boy, blue eyes, curls, a double chin, chubby neck and happy disposition.

"I'm sorry, Mrs. Mack, that you've taken offense but my staff only try and protect me. We do get busy. There are only five doctors to look after 12,000 people."

"Don't start making excuses to me, especially with Johnny so sick."

"OK, Mrs. Mack, we always try to do our best."

"Don't be so condescending, Doctor. Johnny is our only boy, the apple of our eye."

"I understand."

"I don't think you do, Doctor. I don't like your attitude and your tone."

Just then the charge nurse comes in. She's agitated.

"Doctor come quickly. Johnny's pulse and respirations are increasing. He's getting blue and his chest is caving in. He can't get air. Dr. Jim is nowhere to be found."

"Increase the oxygen. Get the set of children's endo-tracheal tubes and laryngoscope. Call the surgeon. I'll be right there. Mrs. Mack, there is an emergency with Johnny, I'll answer the call if that's OK with you."

"Yes, I guess so," said Mrs. Mack.

"If anything goes wrong we'll hold you responsible," added her husband.

Wonderful, I thought.

"OK, let's think of Johnny first. Perhaps you better wait in the visitor's room for now."

I ran to the pediatrics ward and saw Johnny in the croup tent. I heard stridor and saw chest retractions. He was drooling and his skin was blue.

"Tell the parents Johnny is in critical condition," I shouted to the nurse. "Call x-ray and get blood gases. He may have an epiglottis, may have trouble with the intubation. I hope we can get the damn tube in. How's the IV?"

"He'll need a cutdown."

"The surgeon can do the cutdown. I'll have to bag him with pure oxygen and then try and get the tube in. Bring the tracheotomy set."

Here's the x-ray—and Mrs. Mack," said the nurse.

"Oh my god, Doctor, do something," said Mrs. Mack.

"I'm trying, but Billy's larynx, his voice box , is blocked, he can't get any air. I'll try and insert a tube but he may have to have a hole made in his trachea. The surgeon will do the tracheotomy. Here he is now. Please, wait outside."

"I see we have a real emergency," said the surgeon. "Keep bagging him I'll get a cutdown going into his ankle vein. If you can get a an endo-tracheal tube in then I can do the tracheotomy."

"OK. He's not improving with 100% oxygen. Is the IV in? Open it wide. The tracheotomy set is here. OK here we go. His epiglottis is red and swollen. I'm trying to sneak the tube around and through the larynx —there I've got it. You can start the tracheotomy. Jesus, he's still cyanotic."

Johnny gives a cough, the scalpel slips off the midline.

"I'm having trouble bagging him."

"I may have given Johnny a pneumothorax when he coughed. Get x-rays, a chest tube and underwater seal. Keep bagging through the endo-tracheal tube and as I push the tracheal tube in, you slowly withdraw your tube. There we've got the tracheotomy done."

"Here's the chest x-ray. He does have a pneumothorax on the right. I'll put a small chest tube in; now your bagging should be easier. We'll hook it up to an underwater seal," said the surgeon

Billy's pulsimeter rate is slowing and suddenly stops.

"He's no carotid pulse, I'll keep bagging with 100% oxygen. You'll have to start external cardiac massage."

He has no heart beat despite our efforts. Slowly his pupils become fixed and dilated, the cyanosis deepens.

At dawn on a cold, gray November day I declared Johnny Mack dead. I sighed took a deep breath in and went to talk to the parents.

With tears in my eyes, I reached the visitors' room.

"I have bad news, Johnny is dead. I'm so sorry."

"Doc, you let him die," said Mr. Mack as he walked out of the room. "Don't ever speak to me again."

"Oh my God," said Mrs. Mack. "Why did you do this to us, Jesus? Why did you let him die, Doc? My lovely baby is dead." She collapses in the chair and covers her head with her hands.

Three months later, Mrs. Mack phones me to talk over Johnny's death and bring things to closure.

50   I ran into Mr. Mack at meetings in different town and cities. For the next thirty years whenever we met, he refused to shake my hand.

Mello Jello

The phone rings in my office. "Hello, Doctor Haynes speaking."

"Hi, Doc, this is Joe in the coroner's office. I know it's a scorcher and you're busy, and all, but we've got a problem."

"So Joe, what's the problem?"

"The problem is Billy. He's been missing for two weeks. Lives in the apartment next to the medical clinic. Stays in a third floor walk-up above Bob's PX."

"His buddies say they haven't seen him for about a fortnight. Doc, I hesitate to tell you this, but there's a bad smell on the third floor. Do you think it could be Billy frying burgers in this heat in his room?"

"I doubt that. What's the next step?"

"Could you take a lunch break with a big cop? We may have to smash Billy's door down. If you get there first, ask the Super to bring an ax."

"You ask the damnedest things, Joe. What a way to spend my lunch hour. I was looking forward to a fruit salad, maybe an iced tea under an air conditioner."

"The constable will meet you at Bob's PX around noon. I'm sorry, Doc."

Noon finds me in Bob's PX looking at the newspapers. A strange smell seems to be coming from the stairwell or maybe the ventilator. A swamp cooler in the corner chugs, then screeches from a loose fan belt and blows enough fetid air to rattle the newspapers. I pick up the local paper and walk over to the clerk.

"Hi Doc, that's a dollar please," said the store clerk

"OK. By the way have you noticed an odour in here?"

"Yeah, Doc, I've been complaining to the Super for over a week. When I open the store at eight there's a bad smell in here. You know like rotten eggs. It's worse than when they blow the stacks at the pulp mill. I put the swamp cooler on and the fans, they help a bit. My boss has had to close the snack bar at the back of the store because of the odour and lack of customers."

"I smell what you mean. Would you mind buzzing the Super, he called us this morning? The policeman should be here any minute from the coroner's office."

"You think somebody died, Doc? You're the coroner aren't you, and you don't look like a happy camper?'

"Yes I'm the alternate to Dr. Smilie, the chief coroner. Have you got an axe around here?"

"You're not going to knock a door down are you? Is it murder, do you think, Doc? I haven't seen Billy for over two weeks. If it's serious, Doc, let me know first. I could get the scoop for the *Daily Sentinel*. There could be fame and money involved."

"Here comes the constable."

"Yeah, its the big young cop, doesn't look like he shaves yet."

Just then the Super arrives with large ring of keys chained to his belt.

"Hi Doc, Constable," said the Super. "My master key turns the lock in Billy's door. It's likely double bolted top and bottom maybe with a chain. We may need gas masks, the smell is worse than the time all the toilets plugged on the second floor last summer."

As we walked up to the third floor the heat and stench were oppressive. The young constable was getting paler with each step. Standing by the door with the master key, I tried the lock. The tumblers turned but the door didn't open.

"You'll have to cut the frame at the top of the door with the ax and see if you can spring the door."

"Doc, since you're the coroner you get to go first," said the Super.

"Thanks. You guys get the door open."

In a few minutes the bolts are broken off the cheap door frame. I swallow, take a deep breath and enter the small bed-sitting room. Empty booze bottles are stacked in the sink with bits of food and dirty dishes. Cockroaches cover the counters and cupboards, flies buzz over everything. Billy is propped up with pillows in his bed, his body blue and distended. Probably died of heart failure, I think. Body fluids have leaked out onto the carpet. The smell of putrefaction is terrible, barely dispersed by a slow moving ceiling fan.

I look at the Super holding his nose. Around the broken door, a strange sortie of faces, Billy's friends, have gathered. Most of the graying, unkempt men are silent. Tears run down the faces of a few. A woman starts to moan and then wail.

I touch Billy's naked belly and semi-solid waves of fluid course down his bare abdomen. His skin comes off in my fingers. The constable hightails it into the bathroom.

"Poor Billy, we loved him," says one of his friends. "Now he's mello jello."

"Get the constable out of the toilet and have him call the funeral home," I say to the super. "Have them send us some help and masks, gowns and a waterproof body bag. They'll do the autopsy at the funeral home."

I went back to my office and called the pathologist.

"Hello Glen, this is the Sterling. We have an elderly man in his apartment at Bob's PX. He's been dead about ten days in this heat, probably from heart failure but I'll get the medical records sent to you. The body is in bad shape but we'll move him to the funeral home for an autopsy, if that's OK. There'll be an investigation."

"Not another," said Glen. "This is the second today. The first guy was in the North Thompson River for about a month. Be sure to tell them to cool him down quickly. I'll let you know the

54   results within a week."

Two weeks later there was an inquest – a refrigerated case of mello jello.

That Monday Morning Shooting

If it had hadn't happened that morning, it probably would never have happened at all.

I was on call and Charlie was sleeping on the stretcher in the emergency room after a night of hallucinations. He was subdued by the police, me and the drug haldol.

His speech was a word salad of Babel. There was no lighthouse to show me the way. Charlie was 'schitzzie' and on speed. When he talked I didn't know what the implications of "the bird is flying up my mother's ass" meant. I did know he hated women and sometimes his mom.

At 9 am I went to the office and opened the filing cabinet and retrieved Charlie's file. A paper clip attached the latest police report – Charlie had tried to burn the CNR passenger train at Chu Chua. The conductor had tried to hold him in the day coach but the teenager was too agile and escaped into the heavy bush. The conductor called the RCMP.

"Geeze, what a day to be looking for a crazy," said the larger of the cops. "We can't do anything 'til the dogs get here. They'll track him, then flush him out. Charlie is small, tough and unpredictable."

"Yeah," said the other cop. "Heard he's a speed freak."

After a day in the snow and the bush the cops found Charlie huddled up under a cedar. They handcuffed him and brought him into the Emerg at the district hospital where he was committed to the psychiatric ward.

Charlie's days in the ward was uneventful. He was withdrawn but occasionally spoke in riddles—

"I'm afraid of mother. When she dies who'll take care of me? I hate her and I love her. I have sexy girls in my head all mixed up with mother. Crazy thoughts are better than the ones about burning things down, I hate trains." Charlie retreats to the corner and curls up into the fetal position and refuses to talk.

In the psych ward Charlie was subdued. On Sunday he told me his head was wound tight with hemp and he needed BC bud or coke to help him unravel his thoughts.

I tried to pacify him with words of love and concern and his family.

I told him, "The rules were no smoking and no street drugs allowed in the hospital."

"Mom hates me too." He then curled up under the bedclothes and refused to talk.

Late Sunday evening the charge-nurse called me at home. "Charlie's left the ward and taken the warm clothes of the man in the next bed and disappeared. Strangely, he's taken a female's ballroom dancing slippers from the occupational therapy room. At supper he said he had to dance at home, and his brain felt light as a feather. I wondered what he meant?"

"Please notify his folks as well as the RCMP," I said.

Riiing, riiing riiing, the telephone awakened me Monday at 6am.

"Hi Doc, it's me, Sergeant Dan, at the police office. Charlie just waltzed in to his mom's place. There might be trouble, Charlie's taken a shotgun and shells out of the gun cabinet. His dad phoned, said he was talking nonsense."

"OK Dan I'll be right up to the police office after I pick up my bag and drugs. I'll need three constables to go with me; one will have to be backup. No sirens, please. Charlie is very fragile. I'll try to talk to him and defuse the situation."

As we entered the acreage of Charlie's parents we heard a shotgun blast. The picture window, a favorite of his mother's, had been blown out. Then there was silence.

"We'll creep in the back way," I said. "I've known Charlie for ten years. I'll have the best chance of getting the gun. I'll need you after I get the gun."

Slowly we crept into the living room and there was Charlie curled up on the sofa.

"Hi Doc, was expecting you. Didn't hurt nobody, just made a big noise and a hell of a mess. Mom and Dad are holed up in the root cellar. Take the gun, but nobody touches me. Have you got a shot for me now? "He laughs hysterically. "Been shooting heroin all night. No touching now, Doc, OK."

In order to give the drugs, Charlie is held by the policemen. He explodes and rips the tunic from one and the Sam Brown from the other. Eventually he's cuffed and I can administer the IV drugs.

"But Doc, Doc, Doc, you promised, you promised."

What is going on in Charlie's mind is imaginary influenced by a cornucopia of drugs. But who really knows, Mondays just aren't predictable.

A Trip on the Trolley in Trendelenberg

It was a slow and dreary evening in the case room, when the ambulance attendants appeared with a young Italian woman on the stretcher. She was in labour with a prolapsed cord between her legs. I remembered her. Her two previous babies had been delivered spontaneously.

"Place her in the head down position and give her a full flow of oxygen, please," I said to the nurse. "I'll start the IV with a large bore needle. Better get Stewart, he's on call for obstetrical emergencies. Please notify the anesthetist and the obstetrician on call."

"OK," said the nurse.

"Mrs. B, the baby's cord—the life line—came down when your bag of waters broke. The cord is lying between your legs. I'm going to put my hand inside you and push the baby's head back up. This will stop the cord from being compressed against the pelvis when you have a labour pain and allow the blood with oxygen to get to the baby. You'll need an operation, a C-section right away. You do understand, Mrs. B?"

"Yes Mister Doctor," said Mrs. B, "an operation."

"The obstetrician and anesthetist are on their way," announced the nurse.

"Good. I'll drape the patient and try to push the head back up while you help Mrs. B on the trip to the OR We'll need portable oxygen and the trolley in the trendelenburg head down position."

"OK, doctor, we're ready to roll. The patient elevator isn't working, so we'll have to ride with the visitors," said the nurse.

Down the hall we went, all 220 pounds of me, half under the drapes, pushing the head back up in time with Mrs. B's anguished labour cries. The elevators were all in use with visitors clustered around the entrances.

"What's that man doing to that woman, Daddy? Is she having a baby, her tummy looks big? Doesn't the man look funny with his head between her legs," said a little girl to her dad.

"Sir," said the nurse. "I think you and your daughter better take another elevator."

Coming out of the elevator and into the operating suites, I spied Stewart ahead of us.

"A prolapsed cord, I'm pushing the head back. Is the anesthetist here?"

"Nope," said Stewart. "Let me check the fetal monitor. As soon as the anesthetist puts her to sleep, I'll get the baby out."

"Mrs. B, this is the specialist that's going to do the operation."

"Yes," panted Mrs. B. "You get me a big healthy boy, Mister Doctors."

The patient was transferred from the trolley to the operating room table. Mrs. B's cries became louder perhaps from the icy metal of the table against her back, maybe from the icy cold solution being swabbed on her front, the labour pains from above or my big fist pushing from below.

"You better hurry, Stewart, I'm getting muscle cramps in my hand and a crick in my neck," I said.

About two minutes later, I felt a sharp knife-like pain in my right index finger as I pushed on the baby's head.

"You can remove your hand now, Sterling," Stewart announced. "The big, pink boy is out."

Pulling out my right hand, I noticed my rubber glove was cut over my right index finger.

To this day I can feel a small neuroma, see a small scar and feel a small degree of numbness in my finger tip. A little discomfort brings back mirth, merriment and memories. I can still picture the little girl by the elevator and hear her words.

"What's that man doing to that woman, Daddy? Is she having a baby, her tummy looks big? Doesn't he look funny with his head between her legs?"

The Treaty Trip

The screech of shunting cars, bells, whistles and the swearing of car knockers were deafening enough. But they were followed by a series of bangs as the cars locked together, one by one. The train was being made up in Edmonton. The smell of smoke and diesel fuel permeated the platform. Our gear was piled on three large hand carts labeled Northern Alberta Railways. We were leaving Edmonton bound for Waterways and Fort McMurray.

"Jeez I hope I haven't forgotten anything, George, especially that universal dental forceps. I'd be lost without that sucker. My dental instructor said, 'once you get hold of that abscessed tooth with those forceps and with those huge meat hooks of yours the tooth's got to give.'"

"You'll make do," said George

I was a third year medical student going on a treaty trip to Great Slave Lake. The group included George, an elderly ophthalmologist, an RCMP corporal and a constable and an x-ray technician. Our purpose was to pay treaty money and try to improve the health of treaty Indians.

I was the dental extractionist and on the lookout for tuberculosis, disease and abscessed teeth.

The two policemen carried their scarlet dress uniforms with them in a special bag. The treaty money was kept in a large steel portable safe. Every Treaty Indian between Fort. McMurray and Hay River would be paid five dollars for the year. Councilors

64   received ten dollars and the chiefs fifteen. But they had to take their "shots," have a chest x-ray and a physical examination first. As a bonus they could have me extract any troublesome tooth, free.

"All aboard, all aboard," the conductor shouted. Jerk-em-along Reynolds, the engineer took up the slack with a vengeance. The bangs were explosions, the jolts knocked us to the hard, velveteen seats as the train gathered speed. At 7 pm we were underway.

"It will be a long trip with that guy at the engine," said George. "I've ridden with Jerk-em-along before. If you're in the upper birth Sterling you'll be holding on to the straps for dear life. We won't sleep much."

It was a rough night and at dawn we rocketed into Waterways.

"Are you awake, George?"

"Didn't sleep a wink, Sterling. Thank God, there's the station."

"Not much to look at, only the dogs and mud in the street".

"We're not staying here long, have to get the Indian Agent to truck the gear and ourselves over to Fort McMurray and get aboard the motor vessel *The Cross Fox*. We should be able to get breakfast at the Chinese cafe across the street."

About 10 am, the Indian Agent arrived to help us but he seemed preoccupied with his paper work.

"Before any services are performed, every Indian man, woman and child has to have their correct name registered with the band number, treaty number and the reserve. The children must also be identified by the band number of their parents.

This must be recorded on five carbon copies on onion-skin paper, for Ottawa," said the Agent.

"Since the birth of the Dionne quints, it must be federal policy to have everything done in with five copies," I said.

"What if we don't have all the information for the Indian agency?" asked George.

"Then no services or money can be given," said the Agent.

"No five bucks?" I asked.

"It's not the money but the principle of the thing," replied the Agent gravely.

"I agree it sure isn't the money," I countered.

"Come on, let's make tracks for the *Cross Fox*," urged George. "Len, the captain, will want to leave this morning."

We all packed into the van and jolted and honked our way over stretches of corduroy road and snarling dogs until we reached the Athabasca River and the *Cross Fox*.

"I can smell her from here, spilled diesel fuel and stale grease. *Pole Cat* seems more apt than *Cross Fox*. Hope the cook doesn't mix the lard and fuel in the galley or worse with the lubricants in the engine room. My stomach can get as noisy as the engines but I don't want to blow up," I said.

We loaded the equipment onto the boat. George and I decided to bunk at the front of the barge which would be pushed upriver by the *Cross Fox*. That way we'd be away from tobacco smoke, diesel fumes and the head on our journey to Fort Chipewyan on Lake Athabasca.

We were soon underway. We would be tying up the next morning at dawn by the school on the reservation.

The sun was coming up as we docked. The Union Jack was flying on the school's flagpole. The two policemen, brilliant in their red dress uniforms, guarded the steel safe. We set up the tables, the portable x-ray unit, generator and dark room. The shy, moccasin-footed Indians began to appear through the river mist and early light.

"Oyez, Oyez, Oyez," shouted the Corporal. "His Majesty King George the Sixth directs me to pay treaty money. This is our law and your treaty. A new crisp five dollar bill for all treaty Indians." He turned to George and me, "Here comes the chief now."

"Oh yeah," said the Chief. "Five dollars for the land, moose, and fish, you guys got it cheap. All we get is a blue bill."

"Take it easy, Chief, you get three crisp five-dollar bills, your councilmen get two bills. The people in Ottawa are generous and, we, the people of Canada, pay for your treaty rights," said the Corporal.

"BS. We get nothing for the land, we'll take the money and get our check-up but we're getting fed up," said the Chief.

"Geez, what a way to start," I said.

"Oh yeah," said George, "we're all at the mercy of the Department of Indian Affairs. Nobody forgets where they buried the hatchet. We better get started, we've got months of it. Here's the medical routine—x-rays, eye examinations, medical—that's you—and the dental extractions at the end of the day. Today we better work through the list of women and children first. If I see any tubercular keratitis of the eye, I'll give you a shout."

The days went by quickly as we moved up the river to Fort Chipewyan. We visited all the reserves and small villages. I saw and recorded unusual cases of TB, cervical scrofula and psoas abscesses. There were always infected teeth to deal with.

I can remember my first case of dental abscesses, seen in a local chief.

"Doc, pull the sucker out, it's killing me. Better take the next tooth as well, just in case. Oh hell, Doc, you'd better take em all."

As we traveled the Athabasca and Slave Rivers, we saw bear, moose, deer, woodland caribou and even bison at dusk when the animals came to drink. The rivers were peaceful, and in the evening George would reminisce about his many years as a missionary and eye specialist in China. He treated cataracts surgically as well as trachoma and deep foreign bodies in the eye. Minor cases were handled by his Chinese assistants. At the end of his career he taught at eye surgery at medical schools in Peking.

By the time we reached Fort Resolution, George was worn out and he opted to return to Edmonton by plane. Eddie, the bush pilot, picked George and the Corporal up at the river shack air terminal to make connections at Yellowknife with CP Air. I continued by barge with the constable and x-ray technician. We visited different isolated hamlets on the south shore of Great Slave Lake.

It didn't seem right without George, but we continued on to

Hay River and the DC-3 that would fly us home.   67

Even now, almost fifty years later, I can see the mist on the river at dawn and the shy Indian people gathering about flag-poles in schoolyards bearing the Union Jack. I can hear the police chant: "Oyez, Oyez, Oyez, Treaty Time."

Funny Money

My father died poor. My legacy was a safety deposit box full of Alberta's Prosperity Certificates. My dad had been a dentist and had received a Master of Dental Surgery degree. He spent a lifetime repairing maxillas, mandibles and fractured zygomas, removing impacted wisdom teeth as well as doing general dentistry. He and the Dean of Dentistry at the University of Alberta were the only two dentists in Edmonton doing this type of work until much later when plastic surgeons started doing it. Dad was one of the first to have a x-ray machine. The wide scattered rays of the cathode tube gave him exfoliative dermatitis of the hands and later lymphatic leukemia.

Horses were plentiful on Alberta farms in the 1920s and 30s. Iron cranks were used to start cars and tractors. Those were hazardous times—if a shod hoof didn't hit your jaw, the kick-back from the crank could strike you in the face during motor start-ups. Facial fractures were common.

In the days before endo-tracheal anesthesia, it was safer to do these facial surgical repairs under local anesthetic. Dad performed surgery at night and I was the teenage assistant. He taught me the anatomy of the head and neck while he did the three-hour surgery. After placing arch wire splints for fractured mandibles,reducing and immobilizing broken maxillas, he was exhausted and the patient was worn out. Dad was usually paid in kind—chickens, sauerkraut, salt pork. Sometimes, if he was unlucky, the farmers paid him with Alberta funny money.

Funny money was produced under Social Credit Premier Bill Aberhart in 1936. Aberhart was a Calgary high school principal and a disciple of God and an English civil engineer, Colonel C.D. Douglas. Bible Bill adopted Douglas' dictates: the A plus B theorem (the producer of goods A would receive less than the cost of goods B).

Bible Bill, citing The Statute of Westminster, declared that Alberta was a sovereign entity and could control credit and pro-duce Alberta currency to pay for all-Alberta made goods (part B of the theorem). These theories were promoted by the farmers of Alberta.

As an election incentive in 1935, Bible Bill promised all adult Albertans twenty-five dollars. It was no wonder the Socreds were elected. Bible Bill put purchasing power in the hands of the people.

The Alberta Treasury Boards (ATBs) were established and funny money put into circulation. A discount of five percent was given by ATBs for goods and services made in Alberta. "What Alberta Makes, Makes Alberta" was the battle cry of the Socreds.

Everything was to be paid for in Prosperity Certificates of one dollar denominations. The kicker was that every time the cer-tificates were cashed, a very small one cent stamp was to be glued to the back of the certificate, which was marked into one hundred small grids. The stamp glue was poor and the bills large. Over time, with flour-and-water depression glue, the stamps and bills developed a patina of flour. As these 'certs' became heavier and heavier, the stamps became loose and straight pins and small gold safety pins were taken from women's lingerie to secure the stamps. After two years, (the declared life of the bill) they could weigh six ounces. As the glue aged, the certificates became brittle and the funny money could break and shower the floor with stamps.

In Edmonton, the money could be cashed in only a few places—the ATB, Alberta liquor stores, the University of Alberta

Tuck Shop and the Army and Navy Department Store. Nobody wanted cracked money that had to be carried in a shoe box or to give change in good Canadian coin. Finally the Supreme Court declared the monetary system illegal.

Part of the money my Dad received for difficult dental surgery remained in his safety deposit box until he died. A reminder from Bible Bill that Dad's skillful work, performed in the dirty thirties, had been paid for with illegal money produced and signed by Aberhart and the Social Credit fundamentalists.

My father never recouped his losses.

Geoffrey

Geoffrey had knocked about in Western Canada for a few years carrying his two brown suitcases that were fastened with leather belts. The 150 pounds sterling he had arrived with had gone. His polo stick and croquet set had been left in a barn at Cooking Lake. When asked why, Geoffrey replied, "I just couldn't manage to stook ten acres of wheat in a few days and left the farm rather hurriedly."

His favorite cricket bat and wooden tennis racquet were always strapped to his scuffed suitcases. I never saw him use them, although the Garneau tennis courts and cricket fields were close by. My father thought they were stage props to emphasize that "the English upper classes still had the upper hand" in the sporting fields in the colonies.

Geoffrey came to our house in the midwinter of 1930. He was a well-educated Englishman, the second son of aristocratic parents. A remittance man, Geoffrey's received cheques from home that ensured that he would never return to England and embarrass the family. Sometimes the money and single malt Scotch whisky would run out, and he'd be forced to drink Dad's Canadian rye and find a job.

Geoffrey had a sense of class and panache. He was a good actor and joined the little theatre in Edmonton. He had a great stage presence and had a marvelous speaking voice. When the leading man at a dress rehearsal developed laryngitis, Geoffrey filled in with skill and alacrity. He fit the part and his handsome profile, accent and stage presence fit Noel Coward's drawing room comedy. He was a hit, a natural thespian.

After a rehearsal of the play, it was discovered that Geoffrey had no place to lodge. My mother, Elizabeth—the director— took Geoffrey under her wing and brought him home. He stayed off and on for four years. Sometimes he slept on the couch in the front room and occasionally on a single cot by the furnace room.

He still possessed his best suit of plus fours, socks and six detachable collars. His common cry was, "Where are those deuced collars buttons and cuff links?"

Whisky and debating filled Geoffrey's time. To be president of the Anti-Prohibitionist League was right up his alley. He knew how to conduct a meeting and to charm the members of the Women's Temperance League. He was great at costume parties but always needed a drink of Scotch to warm the cockles of his heart.

Geoffrey was always carefree and charming. He liked to wear an English rose in his lapel but never felt he was a thorn in the side of the Empire. To avoid economic worry, he kept busy and was always on the look out for women with money.

Finally, mother found him a job with the University of Alberta radio station, CKUA. The radio station was directly across from my mother's office in the Department of Extension. His mellifluous voice and English accent wowed the Edmontonians. Geoffrey eventually found a permanent job as a radio announcer in Grand Prairie and maintained Grand Prairie was only "a $50.00 trip from anywhere."

My mother had employed a live-in baby sitter named May. Mother did not tell May about Geoffrey. During a winter snowstorm, he arrived about midnight from Grande Prairie. He had taken the streetcar from the CNR station to our house. He left his bags in the hall and stretched out on the sofa with his coat over him. His snores awakened May.

She crept down the stairs, unstrapped his cricket bat from his

suitcase, and crept up to the sleeping man. She raised the bat
and clobbered the apparent intruder.

"My God, you've broken my nose," Geoffrey shouted. We all heard the commotion and ran down stairs. My father grabbed a towel and stanched the flow of blood before it stained the Oriental carpet and new chesterfield.

A few days later Geoffrey announced, in muffled tones "that his nose was getting better and the bruising was subsiding." With Dad's help he bought a one way train ticket to Toronto.

A few months later, we received a letter thanking us for a warm four years. Geoffrey was working as a radio announcer for the CBC and had met a wealthy woman of the horsy set. He was looking forward to a life of polo, theatre, Scotch whisky and marital bliss.

The letter contained a cheque for fifty dollars and was signed "with love, Geoffrey."

The Reluctant Physician

Manyberries, Alberta in July, 1948 was hot as hell fire. I had just broken an axle of the entomology survey truck in the sand hills south of town, hitched into town to get the truck towed in, then joined the survey crew in the beer parlour. It didn't look like the truck was going to get fixed anytime soon.

Our meeting place was the bar of the only hotel. The slovenly barkeeper wore a sweatshirt that proclaimed: "Manyberries isn't the end of the world but you can see it from here." Behind the bar was a flyspecked picture of King George the VI and a Union Jack. Perched on the flag was a stuffed albino pheasant with its tail feathers missing.

I returned to Manyberries 47 years later to study the life of Dr. Sam Bartlett. This time I'd done my homework and had a lifetime of general medical practice in Alberta, California, British Columbia and Alabama to guide me. And to make me appreciate what a godsend Dr. Sam been to his adopted country and community.

Dr. Sam was born in Boston in 1875 and graduated from Harvard Medical School in 1899. The only story he told the Manyberries folk about those days was the time he lost an eye playing hockey for Harvard. In 1911, he set up a homestead south of town. The impetus for the journey from his birthplace to rural Alberta remains a mystery.

North of the border Dr. Sam worked in construction at Fort

Steele, BC before labouring with the Lethbridge irrigation project. While working on a threshing crew in Manitoba, he successfully treated a fellow worker who had broken his leg.

In 1910, the lure of the new land brought him to Orion, Alberta, where he pre-empted a half section on Manyberries Creek and erected a dugout shack in the creek bank. This shack, friends reported, was always a mess. Living with the doctor were pigs, his pet boar JoJo, cats and horses. According to his closest neighbor, Barney Gogolinski, he always kept up with his magazines: *The Harvard Medical Journal, Liberty, Saturday Evening Post* and *The Atlantic Monthly.*

From reading his medical journal, Dr. Sam must have known of the work of Doctor Ricketts and Kin, who, in 1906 and 1907, identified the rickettsia that caused Rocky Mountain Spotted Fever. It was transmitted by the wood tick endemic in the Bitterroot Valley in Montana. Many other clinicians in this region described the virulent form of spotted fever and its high mortality rate. The first was Major W.W.Wood. Later, eight Idaho doctors reported their findings to the Surgeon General of the US.Army.

Dr. Sam corresponded with his sister Madeline A. Bartlett, but no one in Manyberries remembers him traveling east or receiving visits from Massachusetts friends, family or classmates. My research led me to Dr. Sam's father, Dr. George P. Bartlett, an intellectual.

Dr. George Bartlett graduated from Tufts University at age fourteen and subsequently attended dentistry and medical school at Harvard. He was described in a Harvard university publication as a pleasant, well mannered man and an excellent surgeon. Unfortunately he died suddenly of meningitis less than a year after the graduation of his son from medical school. It may have been his father's death that caused the younger Bartlett to give up medicine at his father's sanitarium and seek a much different life in southern Alberta.

The one thing Dr. Bartlett did maintain from the past was a distinct Boston accent combined with a large vocabulary evidenced during his officiating at local town meeting. Barney Gogolinski recalled how 'the Doc' always abided by Robert's Rules. At the first meeting, the Doc talked about the "ex-officio members" having a say. Apparently no one in the community knew what he meant, but the Doc soon taught them.

His patients said that their doctor was very meticulous during midwifery and minor surgery as well as being very fussy in his reduction of fractures. The fractures were immobilized with narrow slats of applebox wood tied together. Dr. Bartlett also pulled teeth. Lawrence Biestefeld remembered "I had a toothache and wanted Doc to pull it, he worked on it for half a day and could not extract it. For ten years I had the same tooth but no more toothache."

During the world-wide flu epidemic of 1918-19, he toiled ceaselessly and dispensed quinine with a lavish hand. In his efforts, Dr. Bartlett was ably assisted by nurses and volunteers. There were very few deaths. Dr. Bartlett even consented to be licensed to practice medicine in Alberta during these years, a licence he never renewed.

After the epidemic, Dr. Bartlett declined offers to practice at the Medical Arts Clinic in The Hat (Medicine Hat) Alberta. Instead he was content to garden, grow watermelon by the wagonload and care for his many cats.

Dr. Bartlett moved from his dugout shortly after some neighbors, inhabiting a similar structure, died of carbon monoxide poisoning when a freak snowstorm covered the chimney and door. He settled in Orion, which meant losing his homestead, but the people of the district built him a small house. With this house, his magazines and his medical practice, he appeared to be a contented bachelor.

In Manyberries and Orion, his habits were accepted, his eccentricities tolerated. He was said to have a shifty look, as he had only partial sight in his injured eye. Apparently the local kids were frightened of his bad eye, ragged beard , bib overalls, and serious demeanor, but most of the local adults didn't think of him as shifty.

It was common lore that the Doc loved to chew snoose. Since his patients knew of his passion, he didn't ever have to buy any. With a large pinch, three fingers and a thumb, he could empty a box. His appetite was only surpassed by his olfactory senses. It was rumored he could smell bread baking a mile away. After a large meal, he was not above criticizing the cook's efforts in a good-natured fashion.

Dr. Bartlett was a frequent presence at many dinner tables since he rarely accepted money for his medical services. He was paid in kind: meals, beer, beef. One old timer remembers a dinner that the Doc ate with a group of men. During an argument over a card game, which distracted the other guests, Doc consumed the entire meal of cabbage and sausage casserole.

The Doc was a long distance walker. Between the scarlet fever epidemics between 1937 and 1942, he was kept on his feet. On one occasion, Dr. Bartlett walked the Black and White trail to Medicine Hat, a distance of eighty kilometers, to obtain a supply of sulpha for four ill children of the town. With prairie winds, dust and dramatic changes in temperature, the trip would have been arduous for a man in his sixties.

In the early 1930s The *Manyberries Chinook* reported his visit to Medicine Hat to have surgery for a strangulated hernia. This event signaled a permanent change in his garb, one most likely recommended by the doctor on the Medical Arts Clinic. When he returned, Dr. Sam was suitably dressed in shirt, tie, jacket and trousers, but not suitably washed.

His failure to bathe and his aforementioned fondness for snoose made him a somewhat pungent dance partner. But despite his odour and difficulty in finding partners, he continued to show up at community dances where he moved with considerable vigor.

At the instigation of Mrs. L. Larson, a widow whose husband died of Rocky Mountain Spotted Fever in 1936, Dr. Bartlett, with local public health officials, developed a vaccination program for spotted fever. Soon after he established spotted fever clinics assisted by townspeople, nurses and government doctors.

A crude vaccine was concocted of infected ticks attenuated with phenol. This was injected three times a year beginning at age three months. Dr. Sam also assisted in the inoculation program for diphtheria and vaccination for smallpox.

In 1953, his Orion shack caught fire, and the Doc was taken to Medicine Hat in burn shock. After a slow recovery, he spent winters in the Hat and summers in a newly built Orion house where he worked in his garden and was looked after by the Farm Women's Institute. These politically and socially minded women made sure everyone was looked after. Those without were given food, shelter, friendship and a place in the community. Apparently Doc was their baby.

Dr. Sam died on Nov. 10, 1956. The Medical Association of Medicine Hat had a granite field boulder brought into the Hillside Cemetery as a gravestone. This stone erratic still marks the grave of one of Albert's most eccentric and caring doctors.

(I'm indebted to the townspeople of Manyberries and Orion for helping me in researching the life of Dr. Sam. My deep gratitude to Barney Gogolinski for taking me around the area and showing me places where Dr. Bartlett lived and practiced medicine.)

PART TWO

AROUND THE WORLD

Black and White

It was hot and muggy just before the rains in Katsina province, Nigeria in1952.

The Fulani tribesmen were gathering with their large horned, humped back cattle and their magnificent steeds.

This was a time of African pomp and ceremony in front of British governors, senior colonial officers and working administrators. Fulanis rode Arab mounts. Chain mail and trappings copied from the Crusades draped horse and rider. Here were the infidels, on sweaty horses, performing make-believe battle charges.

Sultans and chiefs were decked out in their finery by their tents. Hausa traders wore simple long white dresses, red fezzes on their head and lined the perimeter.

Colonial officers were dressed up in uniforms and polished boots. Sweat dripped from us, stained our khakis. French foreign legionnaires from Fort Lamy in Equatorial Africa were present. The meeting was spectacular for me, a Canadian, posted to the south edge of the Sahara in black Africa.

A few weeks later, hundreds of miles away, I was asked by the native chiefs to attend a Fulani native beating in Bauchi province. This was no less spectacular with the pageantry and drums as young Nigerian men administered beatings to their peers. With naked pomp, ceremony and blood these adolescents whipped themselves into manhood with bamboo whips.

86

Both these events have never left my mind. When I left Canada, in 1980 to practice in rural Alabama, I entered another world of American whites and African-Americans.

There was violence in some communities. Shooting, stabbing and knifings were common. In Alabama on a late Saturday night, one of the most dangerous places you could be was in the emergency room of a county hospital. I had a rule that no patient could be seen who had a pistol in his belt or a concealed knife strapped to his leg. 'Nam war veterans sometimes arrived dressed in old battle dress. Many were forgotten addicts, wounded warriors, cast adrift by southern society.

I made many good friends in western Alabama, both black and white, many more than I made in British colonial Africa. Here are some of my stories.

Fulani Beating

Boomlay, boomlay, b-o-o-m-l-a-y, boom.

It's dawn in Bauchi Province, Northern Nigeria. The night drums are slowing and sleepy. The sun is rising and the call to prayers echoes through the savanna country. The worshipping of Allah stops the drums until the morning prayers are over. I was a Colonial officer sympathetic to the rights of the Fulani. The chiefs asked me to attend the young men's rites of passage.

Today is the day of the Fulani beatings. Slowly, the drums reverberate. The beat changes to a charged rhythm. The speed of the beat increases; the large horned humped-backed cattle paw at the dusty ground.

The boy herdsmen are naked, their skins gleaming in the sun. They herd the cattle with long spears. Some of the boys are milking the cows; some are collecting blood from the cattle's neck veins with a sharpened quill. There is blood and milk, food for the young warriors.

The sun clears the horizon. The morning dew has contained the red dust for now. Today will be hot and sultry. There is a lull. The bush dogs and young herdsmen with spears survey the scene. Boys stand on one leg, stork-like, and watch the cattle.

The drums sound lower, the rhythm increases. The chiefs and witch doctors appear in their lion skins. Each wears a head-dress—half-mask, half-hat. Spectators in white robes and red fezzes surround the field.

88   The drummers appear from the grass hut banging out unison. Young males wait to come to centre stage. Young unmarried females appear in their leather skirts, bangles, bracelets and paint. Their plaited hair, their bracelets jingle as they bob in time with the drumbeat. These Fulani women, black Arabs with high cheekbones and aquiline noses are in high spirits, waiting to spur on their favorites.

Suddenly the lean, shiny young men emerge from the huts. They wear leather breech-clouts, their hair and bodies are anointed with butter. Their faces are painted – blue, yellow and vermilion.

The drums reach a crescendo.

The young men dance and leap. Swish of cane whip, boom of the drum, thud of foot. Movements synchronized. Each holds a small mirror in which they watch a gleaming adversary. The mirror shows sardonic expressions, an arrogant stance. There will be no shrieking or calling from pain.

Boomlay-boomlay-boomlay-boom. Thud and s-w-i-s-h in time with the tempo.

Facial grimaces etched, each warrior circles his opponent. S-w-i-s-h, s-w-i-s-h. The two strike each other on the back and flank with the cane in time to the drum beat.

Blood spurts from welts but slowly congeals with grease and dust. The set grin reflected in each mirror never changes—unless the warrior falls from exhaustion, blood loss or death.

They display no emotion, pain or discomfort. The grin reflected in the mirror never changes. The warriors have come of age. They have entered manhood. They can endure.

The witch doctors enter to bind their wounds. Each new adult is rewarded with a calabash of milk and blood. Their badges of courage imprinted on backs and flanks for all to see.

Bloody Practice

The killing of George Washington

Few people know George Washington bled to death. The instrument used was a phlebotome, a spring-loaded lancet three inches long. There was no presidential assassin on the scene, only well meaning bloodletters.

Washington, a large and robust plantation owner, spent all of December 13, 1799 riding his horse in the rain and developed hoarseness and acute croup, then termed cyanche trachealis.

Washington's first bleeding was done by Albin Rawlings, an overseer and clerk at Mount Vernon, Washington's Virginia home. The second and third bleedings were done by a friend, Dr. James Craik. The final bleeding on December 14, 1799, performed by Doctors Elisha Dick and Gustavus Brown, killed Washington. William Cobbett, a contemporary of Washington's and a staunch critic of bloodletting, later estimated that the four bleedings emptied nine pints of blood from Washington— about 80% of his circulating blood volume.[1]

At the time of Washington's death, bleeding combined with purging had been used as a method of treatment for over 2000 years. In 25 BC Rome, Cornelius Celsus made the following statement in his text of early medicine: "to let blood by incising a vein is no novelty; what is novel is that there should be scarcely any malady in which blood may not be let."[2]

In general, bloodletting was either done by venesection (cutting the vein), arteriotomy (cutting the artery) or scarification (shallow cutting of the skin), combined with wet cupping or leeches. The etymology of certain words signals the widespread acceptance of this medical practice. In fact the word leech is a derivative from laech, an Anglo-Saxon word for healer.[3] Methods for removing blood were most likely brought to Britain by the Romans before 450 AD.[4]

Bleeding was used not only for removing "bad blood" but also to ensure optimal vigor. An old English adage pronounces "a bleeding in spring is physic for a king."[5]

Dr. William Harvey, famous English physician to James the First and later Charles the First, advocated bleeding of people to the point of fainting. Even his discovery of the circulation of blood in 1628 did not alter his support for bloodletting. Among his medical recommendations, some of which read like punishments, is the treatment of gonorrhea in men by applying leeches to the swollen scrotum.

In wet cupping, a practice which survived from the16th to the 20th century, the skin was cut many times, and a glass horn, brass or pewter cup was heated, by open flame, and placed over the shallow wounds. Thus a vacuum was created in the cooling cup and the blood was sucked into it.

Failing that, the practitioner could suck the blood from the wounds with a cow's horn, hollow and open at both ends. The narrow end of the horn was then sealed with wax. Usually three to five ounces of blood was removed with each cupping.

In 1834, Dr. W.A. Gillespie, a Virginia physician, advocated use of polished cow horn cups to replace the easily broken glass cups. In 1823, the lancet was the most common medical instrument. At this time, Thomas Wakeley first published the prestigious English medical journal, The Lancet. Thankfully, pointed and cutting editorials in leading medical journals have been instrumental in stopping the use of the fleam and the spring lancet in the twentieth century.

The Smithsonian Institute in Washington, D.C. contains a great collection of bloodletting instruments, lancets and scarificators. These instruments act as silent witnesses to past and present medical practices. The Smithsonian exhibit features a contemporary cow's horn from Madoria, Niger Republic, West Africa. In the 1960s, white missionaries reported bloodletting in the markets of West Africa, where Africans were 'cupped' using horns and razor blades for scarification of their backs and necks.[6]

As a physician, I'd noticed scars on the lower back and buttocks of European immigrants living in rural British Columbia. None of my patients could tell me if the scars were treatment for a specific malady or given to assure continued good health. Some seemed reticent to talk about the ancient customs of their healers.

Then, as now, the practice of bloodletting is carried on without scientific rationale. In fact the persistence of this ancient practice defies logic. While there are certain medical conditions where bloodletting and the use of leeches is beneficial, these are rare.

In North America and Europe, "hematomania" was all-encompassing from the 16th to the 19th centuries.[7] It was pro-

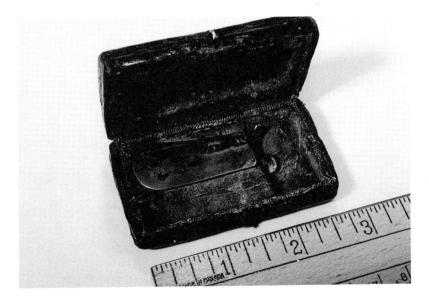

Spring-loaded lancet - similar to one used to bleed George Washington, about 1780. Photo from author's collection

92 moted in the U.S.A. by Benjamin Rush, Josiah Bartlett, Matthew Thornton, Lyman Hall and Oliver Walcott, all medical men, signers of the Declaration of Independence.[8] There were many physicians who opposed bloodletting, but the journalist William Cobbett and Thomas Jefferson were the most instrumental in stopping the practice.

This catchy couplet by Cobett sums up his stance: "The times are ominous indeed /When quack to quack cries purge and bleed."[9]

Perhaps if Thomas Jefferson and William Cobett had been taken more seriously by the medical fraternity, the tragic purging and bleeding of the United States' first president would not have occurred.

1 Davies, Davies and Sanders. William Cobett, *Benjamin Rush and the Death of George Washington.* J.A.M.A. 2, 28, 1983. Volume 249 #7, p. 912-915.

2 Bloodletting instruments in the National Museum of History and Technology, 1979, Smithsonian Institutional Press, Washington, V, 103

3 Avery Jones, Sir Francis. The evolutions of surgery in an English city, *Annals of the Royal College of Surgeons of England*, 1976, Vol. 58.

4 Kuriyama, S. Interpreting the *History of Bloodletting*, The Journal of the History of Medicine and Allied Services Inc., 1995, Vol. 50.

5 Turk, J.L., Allen, E. *Bleeding and cupping.* Annals of the Royal College of Surgeons of England 1983, Vol 65.

6 Bloodletting instruments in the National Museum of History and Technology, 1979.

7 Abel, A.L. *Blood Letting.* JAMA, Nov. 2, 1970, Vol 214, No. 5.

8 Radbull, S.M. *Thomas Jefferson and the Doctors,* Annual lecture in Medical History, Alpha Omega Alpha, University of Virginia School of Medicine, Charlottesville, Virginia, Nov. 4, 1968.

9 William Cobett, *Benjamin Rush and the death of George Washington,* JAMA, Feb.18, 1983, Vol. 249, #7.

Goofer Dust

Three hundred years ago, seventeenth century black slaves arrived from Africa. Their English slavers deposited them onto the coastal islands of Georgia and South Carolina. The people were mostly Yoruba from Western Nigeria and worshipped the Ifa religion. The white planters enslaved them to work in the malaria-infected swamps. They picked cotton, grew indigo and produced rice on island plantations. Their life was influenced by Ifa and their language, Gullah, a blend of various African languages and Elizabethan English. Gullah was woven into work songs and spirituals that sent messages of secret meetings, hexes, haunts and voodoo practices.

After the American Civil War the Emancipation Proclamation gave the Gullah people freedom and some land but not the forty acres and a mule they were promised. They have lived in tranquil island isolation until the developers built the beach resorts in Hilton Head in 1958.

The patent medicine industry was developed in England in the 1700s. One hundred and fifty years later, the industry spread to North America, mainly south of the Mason-Dixon line. African-American folk magic and the herbal medicine of the Gullah paralleled the development of the patent medicine industry and bloodletting used by white doctors and healers.

Andral Kilmer MD graduated from a Chicago medical school in 1865. Dr. Kilmer then perfected his swamp root medicine. He

94 promoted it in newspapers and magazines. Swamp root contained wintergreen, rhubarb extract, mandrake, aloe, juniper, sassafras plus turpentine and other herbs in a 10.5% alcohol base. He enlisted southern American women, "moms" to administer this multi-ingredient concoction to their families for kidney ailment, constipation, influenza and "impure blood." Aggressive marketing and traveling medicine shows promoted Dr. Kilmer's swamp root as well as other products: Lydia Pinkham's vegetable compound (in 15% alcohol), kickapoo oil (in an ether base), fatoff, and perfect headache powders to name a few. They could cure "marasmic disability," "brain fatigue," "torpid liver" and "sick headaches." Pinkham's pink pills were targeted for pale women. Samson's liniment could purportedly knock out pain and Dr. Bell's anti-pain drops were "efficacious" (probably because they contained 9 grains of chloroform and 1.5 grains of opium per ounce).

The patent medicine industry was successful in Canada and the US Dr. Kilmer's nephew, Willis Kilmer, took over the business in 1912. When asked what swamp root was good for Will Kilmer replied, "about a million dollars a year."

Patent medicines became as common as weeds and were unregulated in the US until 1938. Then US president Franklin Delano Roosevelt brought in the Federal Food, Drug and Cosmetic Act. Today patent medicines are regulated although still promoted by testimonials and "satisfied customers."

The Gullah doctors, root doctors, are successful in promoting—by word of mouth—herbs, hexes, canned "jinx killers" and "John the Conqueror's Peaceful Indian Incense," a house blessing for the lovelorn.

Root doctors also practice psychology based on African Ifa religious spells and beliefs. The chewing of certain roots and the sacrifice of small animals and birds sometime will effect a cure. A tortured life or violent death can give rise to restless spirits. In the Gullah lexicon, "trabblin spirits," ghost spirits, can condemn the hexed to an eternity of unrest and madness. The oppressed may be so jinxed by spiritual evil that unless goofer dust is obtained, the hexed could be driven mad. Only goofer dust, taken from grave soil above the heart of a conjure man in a cemetery at midnight, is acceptable. Conjure bags are said to contain goofer dust, buzzard bones, herbs and dolls.

In ancient times "conjuration" by slave doctors was performed. In modern times "conjuration" is performed by Gullah doctors, notably—Dr. Buzzard, Dr. Bug and Dr. Snake. During World War II, Dr. Bug supplied Gullah U.S.army draftees with herbal medicine that affected their hearts. This medicine was taken before the draftees were examined by U.S. army doctors. This native herb caused heart irregularities and abnormal heart rhythms, making inductees ineligible for the draft. I suspect the medicine contained rhodotoxin, a poison obtained from rhododendrons and mountain laurel that causes arrhythmia and even complete heart block.

When one of the Gullah draftees died during the medical examination, Dr. Bug was charged. He was convicted in the state of South Carolina of practicing medicine without a licence and paid a large fine. Then he was nabbed by tax inspectors and convicted of income tax evasion. A few months later Dr. Bug died, a broken man, convinced he had been hexed.

Dr. Buzzard was alleged by the sheriff of Beaufort, South Carolina to have supplied potions in the draft avoidance matter. No one would testify against him, however.

Today, near Sheldon, South Carolina is an independent nation of nine acres, "the Kingdom of Oyotunji." Here, the people still engage in Yoruba Ifa religious practices and tribal marks may be tattooed on the faces of some of the 170 inhabitants. When you enter this village there is a posted sign on the gate proclaiming: "you are now leaving the United States and entering a Yoruba Kingdom. Please leave all your American hexes, spirits and ghosts at the border gate. AMEN."

Swing Low, Dr. D.

The bells were tolling at the white Methodist church in rural Alabama. Dr. D. had died in his sleep.

I mourned him as a friend and a colleague. I was new to the area, a Canadian doctor, recently relocated, and he offered me a genuine friendship. We established our rituals: lunch every Thursday and breakfasts on Sunday.

It was on these Sunday morning breakfasts that he recalled old times. We sat in the small cafeteria of the hospital. Over grits, biscuits and coffee, Dr. D. relived the most exciting time of his life when, in World War II, he served with General Chenault and his flying tigers in Burma. "I can remember how proud I was to patch our wounded pilots as they bounced down the runway all shot up after an air sortie on the Burma Road," he would reminisce. "You know I was the only surgeon. Me, a country boy from the black belt!"

On the other side of the counter, Gloria and Rose, the cooks, shared all their strength in their large bodies, with staff and patients alike, in the form of ample Southern breakfasts and spirituals. "Amazing Grace" and "Swing Low, Sweet Chariot" provided a fitting musical background for Dr. D.'s war stories. Exhausted from emergency room duty, I inhaled the food and talk of adventure.

It rained hard Saturday night, so Sunday morning was hot and steamy. The five pallbearers and I met at 10:30 am in the large wooden vestibule. Shorty, the head pallbearer, gave us all red carnations. The burnished stainless steel casket shone brighter than the summer sun, brighter than the jewels decorating Dr. D.'s daughters, nieces and cousins.

Outside, large Cadillacs and Oldsmobiles sporting New York and Michigan license plates lined the red clay road. Despite the ceiling fans in the church, the men sweated in their dark blue suits and methodically chewed tobacco. Many carried styrofoam cups as spittoons. Their wives dabbed at their eyes clouded with tears, running mascara, and adjusted their mink stoles.

The family wished this to be a segregated affair. The African-American women and children remained outside the church, starting their ceremony by singing in harmony, "We are climbing, Jacob's Ladder," a tune Dr. D. often hummed. Gloria's voice led the chorus and punctuated each hymn with a "We love you, Dr. D., Hallelujah."

"Jeeze, it's hot," I said, pulling at my tie. "Have any of you tried to lift that casket?" The others shook their heads. I thought about Dr. D's last visit to me. According to my nurse, he weighed in at 250 pounds. He loved to eat those massive Sunday breakfasts. We'd be having one now if he were still alive.

"It looks heavy," said Shorty, eyeing the ornamentation on the metal of the casket. "This must be your first southern funeral, huh, Doc?" He winked at me, "if you stay here long enough, the Methodists will get you if the Baptists don't."

With the boom of the organ, six good and true men slowly marched two-by-two toward the casket at the front of the church. As I was the lead pivot man, I had to circle the casket and take the first handle with my left hand. Even before lifting it, I started to envy the three men using their right.

The sermon began slowly, the preacher stretching his words to fit the wide shape of this man. He paused frequently and droned on, oblivious to heat, time, or the buzzing of flies. I let the words slide by, but watched for him to signal us forward.

Shorty whispered, "This is it, boys, one quick lift and slow step it to the limo."

I wondered if we could do anything else.

Veins in our hands, faces and necks stood out. We slowly marched out the centre aisle, trying not to grimace. I pictured Dr. D. laughing at our efforts, but pitying our plight. I imagined him chortling, "You know, boys, I wouldn't have et all those plates of grits and butter if I'd known you'd be so hot and I'd be so heavy."

To get the casket into the hearse took an extra heave onto the rollers. The springs on the Lincoln sank lower and lower as we slid the casket in.

"Wipe yourselves off, Boys," said Shorty. "It will be tougher at the cemetery. This time of year, that red clay is bound to be slippery."

Gloria, the lead, had started singing again, the rest of the women harmonizing. But the hymns seemed faster, with a syncopated beat. Hands clapped, braided corn-rows bounced, and patent leather shoes kept time as the children followed the mourners to the burial grounds. We walked past the massive redwood tree, past the graves of three hundred Confederate soldiers who had died 140 years ago at a makeshift hospital in town. The air felt heavy, the ground gummy.

"All them high heels is going to take a beating in this mud," said Shorty, falling in step with me.

"We're going to take a beating too," I said.

Shorty sighed, "I sure hope Dr. D. 'preciates this," then added. "I could sure do with a co'cola."

Plowing mud, the hearse beat us to the prepared grave site.

Shorty pointed to the site, "Just as I expected. Only three four-by-fours across the grave. I hope they hold the casket and Dr. D. We may have to hold the casket with those canvas straps if the timbers give way. Too bad all us pallbearers didn't have a say on the type of casket. Musta been those women from Deetroit who chose it."

With a super human effort we retrieved the casket from the back of the hearse.

A few sliding steps got us to the grave. By digging in our heels we managed to avoid slipping into the hole. The timbers creaked with the weight of their burden.

"Ashes to ashes, dust to dust," the prayer began.

"Where's the dust?" I muttered as we lifted the canvas straps to allow the agile gravediggers to remove the timbers.

"We're on our own boys, hold tight," whispered Shorty. "Keep your ends up. This preacher drawls real slow."

I thought of Dr. D. training at Tulane University in the lazy heat of the Mississippi River and then freezing in Minnesota during his surgical training. He shared case after case with me, a woman in prolonged obstructed labour, Dr. D. administering the anes-

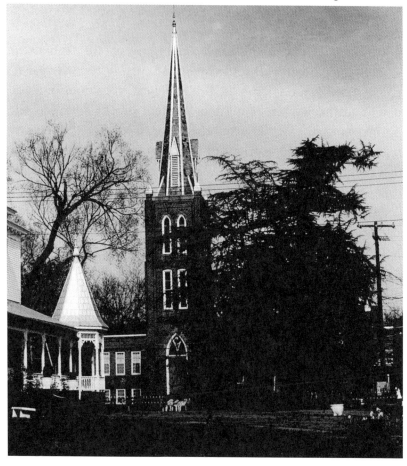

Methodist Church, Marion, Alabama, 1988. Photo from author's collection.

thetic and delivering her son by C-section. He was over six feet tall now and the woman constantly pronounced that Dr. D. was "her goodness and her savior." She wasn't alone in her feelings. Dr. D. lost none of his compassion over the years. As I performed my last act as a pallbearer, I pictured him back with General Chenault, flying as high as he ever would get.

We lowered the casket containing our good friend. Down he went. All gathered to pay their last respects, a flower and some red clay in one hand. Soil and blooms soon covered the casket.

Gloria's full-bodied soprano voice led the mourners in song. "Though the road is steep and rugged, though the road is steep and rugged. Though the road is steep and rugged, we are climbing on."

Interviewing Alabama Veterans – a Physician's Perspective

In the South, "What do you know good?" was my patients' usual greeting as they entered my office. As a physician newly arrived from Canada, I found that asking directly about what brought the men to see me was not very successful. They didn't like slick dress, hair or talk. So I soon learned to ask questions such as: "Do you have kids or dogs?" and "Where'd you go to school?" Then I could proceed to: "Were you in 'Nam?' You seem to be limping."

Today, a man appears in the office dressed in an old battle uniform. After the small talk, he says:

"I'm havin' these nightmares, Doc. Sometimes they carry over into morning. The killin', the hollerin', the wounded, the noise. Those land mines everywhere. Those little two-bit plastic mines—I hate 'em, hate 'em. Those mines is diabolical, they can blow off a foot and go up into your privates. I can't get 'em out of my head, the flashbacks over and over, shredded dicks, balls and feet floating in the rice fields. Excuse the language, Doc. I gotta do something, my nerves is shot. You'd snort coke if you was me, Doc. My Gawd, Doc, think on it – no balls and peeing through a hole between your legs. I gets urges, Doc, but it's all in my goddamn head."

Suddenly, he's crying silently. Then sobbing. The interview comes to an end.

The Fires of Venus

In rural Alabama in 1982, we started a venereal disease clinic. It was housed in an old brick building which had a weathered sign saying "VD Clinic." The public health office in Montgomery had renamed it "The Sexually Transmitted Disease Clinic." We never took the original sign down.

We treated people, free of charge, for syphilis, gonorrhea, thrush and trichomonads. We did pap smears and diagnostic testing. We gave out birth control pills, condoms and tried to do family planning for our patients who were poor and uneducated about such matters. Later, we did HIV testing for AIDS.

One rainy afternoon I was stopped by a large African American woman in her forties. She looked sick and sweaty.

Venus, as she quickly introduced herself, asked to be examined immediately. "Hey Doc, I must have 'fireballs' but don't mash me cause I'm hurtin'."

"We'll try and see you as soon as possible, Venus."

"How soon Doc? My private parts been on fire for over a week. I'm all sweated up and I cain't stand Joe, he's my live-in, y' know. Don't think I can stand for you to mash me or use one of them specolums. Doc, please get me in soon."

I agreed to make her a priority. When I finally had her in the examining room, I asked her how many children she had.

"Had six kids with Joe and three with that no 'count Earl. Had some miscarriages too. Guess I been pregnant about a dozen times. Last period was regular about three weeks ago. Don't take birth control pills, but I use the shield. Had it in me for about six years off and on."

"What do you mean by off and on?"

"Them little things kept coming out but I just shoved those lil' bugs back up even if they'd lost the string. Sometimes, if I had the money, I'd go to the Doc and he'd stick a new one up," she explained to me.

I told Venus to get on the table and put her feet in the stirrups. I warned her that I would have to use the speculum.

"Ah's sick, Doc, don't mash me hard," said Venus. She then had me pass her a styrofoam cup so she could spit out her snuff before the examination began in earnest.

"Your lower abdomen is not moving at all. Have you been constipated?" I asked.

"I ain't had a good shit in a week, but where your mashin' me really hurts, Doc."

"I realize you are ill, Venus. You'll have to be admitted to hospital. You have an infection in your tubes. I have to take the IUD out now."

"Doc, Joe and I ain't got no money. President Bush done took me off Medicaid and I owe the hospital $400. Margie, in admitting, won't let me in even if I'm dying. Please treat me with pills."

"I'm going to have to use the speculum and pull the IUD out. I think it's a Dalcon shield, Venus."

"Doc, I hate to lose it, it's been my security."

I asked the nurse for another pair of ovum forceps. I got hold of protruding string but the attached IUD seemed to be stuck. Slowly, I felt it dislodge.

I saw the Dalcon shield reluctantly make an appearance on the speculum. To my horror, a second one appeared to be hooked onto the first one. Then a third shield had leap frogged onto the second shield. The strings had come off the spider legs of the shields and become hitched together.

With each tug, Venus would give a sharp cry.

"That's really hurtin' Doc. Hope you're done."

"I expect that's the lot, Venus. The nurse will give you some pain pills, antibiotic pills and a shot of penicillin. If you get worse, go to the hospital. You can go shortly, but see me tomorrow."

"I sure do 'preciate you helpin' me, Doc. But if I gets pregnant, guess I'll have to blame ya'll."

I Have a Dream

In August, 1963, at the Lincoln Memorial Centre in Washington DC, theologian and social activist, Reverend Martin Luther King, gave his "I have a dream" speech in front of 200,000 people. Here is part of that speech:

I have a dream that one day this nation will rise up and live out the true meaning of its creed. We hold these truths to be self evident, that all men are created equal....I have a dream that one day on the red hills of Georgia, sons of former slaves and sons of former slaveholders will be able to sit down together at the table of brotherhood....I have a dream that one day even the state of Mississippi, a state sweltering with the heat of injustice, will be transformed into an oasis of freedom and justice.[1]

Reverend King's vision of passive resistance and freedom was set in motion in1963. Byron De la Beckwith, a white suprema-cist, assassinated Medgar Evers of the NAACP (National Association for the Advancement of Coloured People) in Jackson, Mississippi.

Protesters complained that white people would not let blacks vote. In Mississippi, black voters were "persuaded" to voluntar-ily remove their names from the voters' list. Supremacists and the Klan were active in Marion and Selma, Alabama where I opened a practice at the Perry clinic. Reverend King's wife, Coretta Scott King, was raised in Marion, Alabama. Her parents, Obie and Bernice Scott, were interesting patients of mine. Through my contact with them and the family, I became interested in the civil rights movement.

Obie and Bernice were honourable folks who ran a grocery store in rural Alabama. They were straightforward, honest people. Obie would phone me for an appointment. He liked to come in early, 9 am If he wasn't seen promptly at nine, he could get impatient. He didn't like leaving the store. It was surprising to me that the store was open most of the time , as Obie was over 90 years old. Obie and Bernice both had serious health problems, but weren't complainers and only appeared when they had a legitimate concerns.

I moved to Marion from BC when the Federal Health Development Corporation recruited me. I looked after the school cadets at the Marion Military Institute (MMI). I also looked after many of the black people of Perry County. We had the first desegregated waiting room in the county. The ice cold water in the fountain was free and we had flush toilets and air conditioning. I had a captive audience, but as there were few telephones in my patients' homes, many of the sick came as drop ins and my waiting room overflowed with patients. I sometimes wondered who was captive? The MMI cadets sent by some of their families for "behaviour management," the ill, the poor with no medical insurance, or me?

Fifteen years before I arrived, the freedom march from Selma to Montgomery took place. At the Pettus Bridge over the Alabama River, Sheriff Clark and Alabama State Troopers under Governor George Wallace stopped 700 black protesters. With tear gas, attack dogs, night sticks and cattle prods, mounted police waded into the crowd beating men, women and children, arresting all. The wounded were taken to the Good Samaritan Hospital in Selma and finally "Bloody Sunday," March 7, 1965, came to an end. A few days later, 300 school children were arrested and jailed for allegedly rioting.

Several weeks before this, 700 black marchers were arrested in Marion's town square beside the Zion Methodist Church. During the melee, a seventeen year old woodcutter, Jimmie Lee Jackson, was shot in the belly by a state trooper. The local doctor refused to attend the victim, and he died in Selma eight days later. That night, the spotlights in the Town Square were shot out by white supremacists and national newspapers had pictures of the police brutality, the night the lights went out in Marion.

Club-swinging state troopers waded into black demonstrators. When they marched out of the church to protest voter registration practices, at least ten people were beaten bloody. Troopers stood by while white bystanders beat up media cameramen. Later, after Reverend James Reeb, a Boston Unitarian was clubbed in Selma and died in hospital, President L. B. Johnson sent in 1800 National Guardsmen to protect the marchers. Finally, in the summer of 1965, the Federal Voting Rights Act was passed in Congress giving black people the right to vote.

When I left Marion nine years after I arrived, Bernice and Obie Scott came to tell me goodbye and "hug my neck." The Scotts lamented my leaving and Obie paid me a great compliment. "Doc, you're the first white man I ever trusted," he said.

1 Part of the "I had a Dream Speech" by Reverend Martin Luther King was taken from the Freeman Institute's publication, 1103 Burkhart Lane, Severn, Maryland, USA

Cuban Medicine

It was Marti day, January 28, 1998 and we joined in the procession which moved from the University of Havana's steep granite steps to the vast Parque Central in old Havana, where it was rumoured Castro might speak. Our wooden sticks wrapped in rags, dipped in kerosene and set alight wobbled dangerously and smoldered as we shouted "Cuba, Cuba, Cuba." We swayed with the crowd, admiring the fashionable Cuban women, ahead of us, dancing to the rumba rhythm. We were singing on the long walk to the square.

"Marti, Marti, Marti," we shouted. We were honouring Jose Marti, the Cuban philosopher and poet as decades of Cubans had done before. Did we honour Fidel Castro, Dr. Che Guevara and the revolution? Grim faced soldiers lined the streets. There would be no rioting. Billboards proclaimed UJC (Union de Jovenes Communista) and PCC (Partido Communista de Cuba).

I was in Cuba to study Spanish, Cuban health care and culture with a group from York University, Ontario. It was difficult to teach me, a deaf old man, Spanish. Classes ended at 3:00 pm, then I could look forward to excursions outside the classroom to hospitals, museums, stadiums, and theatres.

We walked the streets and interacted with the people. The Cubans appeared happy and friendly, but in repose some faces seemed strained and anxious. The US embargo was strangling the people economically but there was a tight noose of government controlled action and thought, soldiers and police were everywhere.

The Russians left Cuba in 1991. There was no gasoline, food was rationed and the Cuban peso worthless. Those lucky enough to have US currency could buy anything. The American dollar was king. Salaries of Cubans were low, a senior teacher received approximately 320 pesos a month (about twenty dollars). Surgeons made about 400 pesos per month. In one hospital, operating rooms had closed because of lack of anesthetic agents and soap. My Spanish teacher's father was an insulin dependent diabetic who was in a diabetic coma because of lack of insulin. Finally, insulin arrived from Canada's Connaught Laboratory to Havana.

The contrast between community medical clinics and Russian built hospitals were enormous. The clinics were busy and well organized. The vaccination programs were better attended and organized than Canada's. Ninety-eight per cent of Cuban children were fully immunized. The educational plan to promote safe water was good. All water had to be boiled for drinking, some bottled water was provided. The sewage system was poor and garbage pickup in the streets sporadic.

The hospital I visited was impressive, built on a grand scale by the Russians. There were fancy elevators, marble walls and terrazzo floors, but there were few patients. I saw no patient with an IV running when I visited the wards. Doctors told me of shortages of insulin, antibiotics, oxygen, anesthetic agents and even bandaging. When asked about the treatment of AIDs patients, the charge nurse said, "AIDs is not a Cuban problem." When I asked the same nurse about the incidence of sickle cell anemia, common in the southern US, she replied that sickle cell anemia was not a problem and only occurred among Africans. I found these answers naive and unbelievable.

We also learned about the work of Dr. Forness and his Cuban band of engineers, sociologists, health care workers and environmentalist who are trying to reclaim Havana's Rio

Alamendares. Badly polluted by sewage and factories, the river is a cesspool as it enters the Gulf of Mexico. Cuban and Canadian environmentalists have defined and mapped pollution problems. I wish them well in their attempts to restore and reclaim this fresh water source. Today purified, treated water is in short supply. Sewage treatment plants are in disrepair.

The streets were full of push-carts, bicycles, old Russian cars, Chevys and Buicks of 1952 to 1956 vintage. The Russian cars were dilapidated but the American cars were running and painted pink and purple. The big tail fins were a reminder of the past, the Mafia, the United Fruit Company and the exploitation of the Cuban people. The ingenuity of the Cuban mechanics keep these cars running. Public transportation is provided by two types of buses, the camel (el camello) and the aspirin (el aspirino). The camel buses were shaped like camels with a hump at each end and resembled modified cattle trucks. They were hauled by old Mack truck tractors. On most days, 400 Cubans could be packed together in each bus. The hump part of the el camello is termed the barbecue, a descriptive term on a hot day. El aspirinos use unleaded gas. They were rough, jammed with people and full of fumes. After a ten kilometer ride, I had a headache and wished for an aspirin. Most Cubans brought their own.

The Cuban medical schools are good. The physicians I spoke to seemed dedicated. The Cuban plastic surgeons must be talented as we saw middle aged gringos, sporting dark glasses, in expensive hotel bars with subdued light. I'm sure the glasses masked the bruising that occurs with face lifts and rhinoplasties. The total cost was said to be about ten percent of the cost of plastic surgery done in New York or Madrid.

The entertainment at the Grand Teatro, a Cuban theatre, was outstanding. The Spanish built the theatre in 1832. The marble floors and walls, the mahogany doors and sparkling chandeliers reflected the opulence of the years of Spanish domination. We saw two performances there: Swan Lake with full orchestra and a modern dance production set in Yoruba country, Nigeria.

116   Both were world class productions.

Canada/Cuban relationships are improving. Tourism is increasing and our understanding of the Cuban culture better. I think Castro is making an effort to improve the human rights of some. I'm not sure if political prisoners are accorded many rights under the present dictatorship. The Cuban people like Canadians, and tourists are safe in Havana streets. I will forever remember our march to Parque Central on Marti day. When our torches went out we linked arms and sang together "Cuba, Cuba, Cuba."

Natural Medicines of Belize

Where is Belize? A Belizean writer, Emory Stephen says "it's south of Paradise and north of Frustration." It borders on Guatemala, Mexico and the Caribbean. What was the British Honduras, became an independent nation of Belize in 1981.

Explorers in an Interhostel group, our group was in Belize to learn about *la ruta Maya*,—the trade, medicinal and war routes taken by the Mayan people for centuries. Belize is swampy, and tropical with epiphytes, flowers and plants as well as millions of anopheles mosquitoes lurking in the jungle. Malaria is prevalent throughout Belize.

Walking down the rainforest medicine trail outside of San Ignacio, I saw a wealth of useful plants and trees that have been collected and used by Dr. Rosita Arvigo. The trail is dedicated to her late Mayan mentor Don Elijio Panti, renowned healer and last Mayan shaman of Belize. The medications are still being collected and used. Their names very descriptive:

1. Bull Horn Acacia: the bark is a partial antidote for snakebite and will give the victim time to get to the hospital for anti-snake venom.

2. Piss the Bed Plant: the extract from this plant can be ingested as a laxative. In small doses is used to treat bed wetting in children.

3. Skunk Root Bush: a tea made from leaves of this bush protects the patient from witchcraft or alcoholism, or both!

I recorded many other medicinal plants described by Dr. Rosita Arvigo in her *Ix Chel* garden. As I made the circuit of the garden I was about to lean against the Black Poison Wood tree but was stopped by our Mayan guide. The bark of this tree is very toxic and in times past Mayan prisoners of war were tied to this tree until their skin fell off. An antidote was an extract obtained from the bark of the nearby Gumbolimbo tree.

A useful tree is the Gumbolimbo tree. I mistakenly called it the Gringolimbo tree at first, because it peels its bark and resembles the pale, peeling sun burnt skin of the Gringo Tourist.

As I left one forest garden a large sign caught my eye:
"HEY MAN—BETTA NOT LITTA."

I wondered if the punishment for littering would be one week tied to a Black Poison Wood tree.

After leaving the Panti medicinal trail, we took a short bus trip from San Ignacio to Xunantunich (pronounced shoo-nahn-too-NEECH) meaning stone maiden. We had to cross the Mopan River in a hand-driven ferry, mechanized by a series of bicycle sprockets and chain. The tourist guide told us that the Mayan ferry operator did not want his picture taken. Many Mayans believe that their spirit is stolen by the camera and may be lost. One tourist insisted on photographing him and was immediately confronted by a Mayan warrior who morphed from the docile ferry operator. I heard the offending film 'splat' when it hit the surface of the water.

We walked to the ruins up the hill. This same track we were walking, in ancient times, controlled riverside travel from Tikal in Guatemala to the Caribbean Sea via the Belize River.

Lining the track were shady ceiba trees, the tree of the Mayan gods, and bull hoof vines intertwined with the spectacular Belizean black orchids. The magnificent bull hoof vine can be sixty meters long and thicker than a wrist. The thick male vine can be chopped up and made into a tea to staunch bleeding internally if drunk or applied externally to skin. The thin thorny female vine can be made into a tea and drunk for birth control. A woman may drink three cups of tea the first three days of her menstrual cycle and she will be infertile for six months. The maximum dose taken every six months can be given for only eighteen months. This contraceptive tea is believed to prevent the implantation of the fertilized egg by changing the uterine lining. The World Health Organization is studying the vines' special effects.

At the top we saw El Castillo, a pyramid rising forty meters above the jungle floor. The silence of the jungle, the heat, the humidity, the stone slabs of writing and the buildings made me feel insignificant. Here was a civilization I had never dreamed existed, Mayan history recorded by Indian hieroglyphics and drawings on stelas.

I could envision *Ixtabai,* a mythical Mayan forest creature described by Dr. Arvigo as "a tall beautiful woman with her feet on backwards, sitting in the branches of the ceiba tree wooing unfaithful husbands to disappear with her into the underworld through the trunk of the ceiba tree."

The Mayan hieroglyphics with 850 symbols have been deciphered. The glyphs show us that Mayan society was complex with aristocracy, pageantry and spirituality. Tales of kings, lords of city states, and pageantry are recorded and dated from their ancient calendars on the newly discovered stelas. Their history has been hammered in stone and we are only now able to break the code.

Dr. William Gorgas and the Building of the Panama Canal

"Beyond the Chagres River
'Tis said—the stories told
Are paths that lead to mountains
Of purest Virgin gold,
But 'tis my firm conviction,
Whatever tales they tell
That beyond the Chagres River
All paths lead straight to hell."
James Stanley Gilbert

The French, American, Chinese and West Indian workers in Panama experienced the Chagres hell first hand. Chinese coolies were so melancholy from disease, rain, mud, and grim working conditions that one night hundreds of men committed suicide en-masse at a place called "matachino" (death of Chinese in Spanish). They jumped off cliffs and impaled themselves on sharpened bamboo sticks below.

About one hundred years later, I cruised past the town of Matachino. The mud and cliffs were still there but the waterways of the Panama Canal were now open. I stood in the oppressive heat, watching massive drag lines and ore trucks take the mud away and thought about how Dr. William Gorgas, eradicator of yellow fever, and the US Corps of Engineers finally got the canal through.

In 1534, Charles the First of Spain ordered the first survey of a proposed canal at the Darian Gap in Panama to follow the Chagres River. The engineering problems were so immense that the plan lay idle for over 300 years. Ferdinand De Lessup, fresh from building the Suez Canal was chosen to build the Panama Canal. Five other routes were considered but De Lessup, the French entrepreneur, and the French Congress chose the one through the Darian Gap along the Chagres River. This route was condemned by leading engineering authorities, notably Baron Godin de Lepinay and Gustav Eiffel. De Lessup proposed a sea-to-sea canal but hadn't considered the Sierra Mountains.

The Rothschilds were the bankers and supported De Lessup. They did not know that Lieutenant Wyse of the French army had not completed the second land survey. The first survey had ended in failure because of death from disease of many of the French engineers. Wyse, an assistant and close relative of De Lessup, produced a map that was inaccurate and was said to have been completed in the bars of Colon, Panama. No one voted for an "open cut canal" initially except the bankers, Wyse, De Lessup, and the French congress.

From 1880 to 1889, the French struggled with disease, corruption, financial and engineering problems. Finally they admitted the mud and disease were too much. Many Frenchmen were dead, the engineering pride of that generation defeated, and the country bankrupt. The Canal was only partly completed, and the equipment in ruins when the work on the Canal was abandoned for almost a decade.

In 1898, the US battleship blew up in the Havana harbour, inciting the Spanish-American War. Soon Teddy Roosevelt and his "roughriders"—US marines—were in Cuba. American troops were dying from malaria, yellow fever, and typhoid. Roosevelt appointed Dr. William Gorgas as medical officer in charge of the marines' health. Dr. Gorgas and his wife were immune to yellow fever as they had contracted it years before when treating epidemics at Florida army bases.

Gorgas and his army partner, Dr. Walter Reed, had studied the works of Dr. Ronald Ross in India. Dr. Ross had discovered the life cycle of plasmodium, the cause of malaria, and knew that the anopheles mosquito transmitted the plasmodium. In 1902 Dr. Ross won the Nobel Prize for his discovery. Doctors Gorgas and Reed realized that the anopheles mosquito laid their eggs in clear fresh water containing grass and algae, but were poor flyers and easily controlled. They agreed with the Cuban physician, Dr. Carlos Findlay, that the mosquito stegomyia fasciata spread yellow fever. Armed with the knowledge of Dr. Ross and the theory of Dr. Findlay, they started their assault on the mosquitoes of Cuba.

Squads of 50 to 150 sanitation workers declared war on all mosquito breeding places. They put screens on rainbarrels, oiled puddles and cesspools, and drained pools. In hospitals, windows were screened and the sick were quarantined. The anopheles brigade cleaned up grasses and algae around ditches.

In 1901, American President McKinley was assassinated and Vice President Teddy Roosevelt took over the presidency. Secretary of War William Taft and Roosevelt took over the building of the Panama Canal. With the US Marines and the US Navy, they forced Colombia to give Panama independence. They bought the Panama Canal land rights from the state of Panama and the French Canal Company for $50,000,000—a bargain. Roosevelt boasted, "I took the isthmus."

Roosevelt and Taft appointed Dr. Gorgas as medical officer and John F. Stevens as chief engineer to take over where the French left off. Stevens was overworked and hassled by Congress and quit in 1907. He was replaced by Major Goethals, chief army engineer. Major Goethals completed the fifty-one mile canal in 1914.

The Major planned a 'lock and dam' approach to building the canal. This was a slow, arduous process. The sanitary engineers under Dr. Gorgas were thwarted by Admiral Walker, a high ranking navy official in Panama. Walker discounted mosquito control as "balderdash." General Davis, the governor of Panama, told Dr. Gorgas "to get that mosquito idea out of your head." Fortunately Dr. Gorgas and Major Goethals persevered with their work, despite the jungle heat, humidity, rain, mud, and rock. The Chinese coolies and the West Indian roustabouts died in untold numbers, but the mortality after 1908 declined mainly because Gorgas had controlled malaria and yellow fever.

After the canal was completed, Dr. Gorgas was posted to South Africa to help with the problem of pneumonia in black miners. Then he assisted the Rockefeller International Health Board and worked in Peru, Ecuador and the Belgium Congo to control malaria, yellow fever and pneumonia.

He was appointed first Surgeon-General of the US Army, knighted by King George the Fifth of England and awarded the Star of Belgium by King Albert. He received a Doctor of Science degree at a special convocation at Oxford University. At a Royal Society meeting in London, Sir William Osler, the renowned Canadian physician, said, "Perhaps of all living Americans, he had conferred the greatest benefit on the human race."

Surgeon-General Gorgas died in England, July 3, 1920. The funeral took place at St. Paul's Cathedral, London, England. Later, he was buried at Arlington National Cemetery, Washington, DC.

I turned to look at the cliffs of Matachino and imagined Dr. Gorgas in rumpled khakis and pith helmet looking down at this waterway. Now boats from all over the world pass, their passengers and crews untroubled by the ravages of malaria and yellow fever.

Medical Emergency in the Canals of Tortuguero

When we arrived at the Pacuare River in Costa Rica our boat, a flat-bottomed scow with a laced canvas roof and an outboard engine was waiting for us. The guide, Pedro, hurried the eight of us aboard with call of, "Vamos, ahora." Our Interhostel group was heading for the canals of Tortuguero, east of San Jose, on the Caribbean, to bird watch and enjoy the jungle flora and fauna.

The captain started the engine and we pushed off. Howler monkeys swung from abandoned cables of defunct banana plantations. A three-toed sloth hung upside down in a tall "tourist tree" by the marina. The red and peeling bark of these gumbolimbo trees resembled the pink skin of sunburned gringos like me.

As we proceeded down the muddy, slow-moving river, the landscape slowly changed, the jungle becoming denser. Two-hundred-foot trees covered with vines, epiphytes and orchids lined the banks of the river. Caimans, their mouths gaping open, basked on logs in the sunlight. We photographed the roseate spoonbills and white ibises. The bird chatter was incessant.

After miles of river, we turned into a tributary. We had arrived in the Canals of Tortuguero. It became much hotter and the humidity was oppressive. The captain geared down to push masses of purple-flowered water hyacinth out of our path.

Slowly, we inched past a dredge mired in muck and weeds and could smell the sweetness of decay. The captain managed to wiggle the boat through to an eddy where other scows were waiting for us to pass. These boats were smaller and filled with binocular- and camera-toting naturalists. Around a tight bend, we spotted the Jesus Christo iguana, its huge flat toes and feet splashing the water surface as it propelled itself across the lagoon.

Beyond the lagoon was the fishing camp, Parismina Tarpon Rancho, our destination for lunch. I noticed two guards with AK-47 assault rifles on the pier, their presence belying the peace of the place. They were there ostensibly to protect the gringos from bandits who lived in the area.

The fishing camp boasted an "all you can eat" lunch. As we entered the café, I saw a man sitting with his head cradled in his hands. A terrible hangover, I wondered? Too much food or sun? We were waiting for our food to arrive when a guide approached our table and asked, "Is there a medical doctor here?"

I obligingly answered yes, hoping I wouldn't be needed for something serious like a heart attack or drowning. I had retired from my practice a couple of years ago and felt rusty.

Slumped on a bench was a tall, muscular white-haired American, his problem obviously not being resolved by the glass of warm milk being proffered by a guide.

The man looked up at me and said, "Who the f… are you and who is this SOB trying to feed me milk?" He warned, "Don't you try to get into the act."

I sat down on the bench beside him and said, "Do you have any medical problems?"

"None of your f…ing business. Who the hell are you?"

"I'm a retired Canadian doctor. Thought you might have a problem. I noticed a bracelet on your wrist."

"None of your goddamned business, Doc," he said. "And don't you try to get me to eat. Didn't eat supper and didn't feel like eating breakfast."

"Did you take insulin this morning?" I asked.

"Your damn right I did and last night, too, but I ran out of candy bars. Or maybe I forgot."

He seemed to be getting shaky. I took his pulse. It was fast. His face looked sweaty and his speech was slurred.

"Keep your f…ing hands off me, Doc. There's nothing wrong with me."

"Quick, get me a large glass of water and put five to six table-spoons of sugar in it," I said to the guide. "He's having a serious reaction from too much insulin, his blood sugar is probably very low. He likely hasn't eaten any food for eighteen hours but has taken at least two doses of insulin. Put two straws in the glass."

"No straws out here," he replied.

"Just get me the water."

He brought the sugar water, and I persuaded the man to take five or six big swallows of it. Finally, with much resistance, he drank the whole glass.

Suddenly, his demeanor changed. "What's happening?" he asked.

"You were getting rather agitated," I replied.

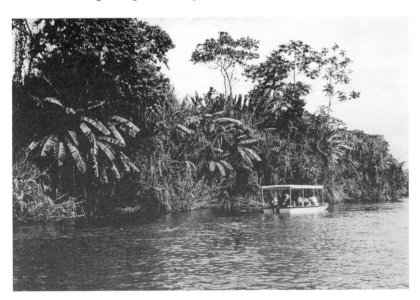

Canals of Tortugera. Photo from author's collection.

"Did I say anything mean or ugly?" he asked.

I smiled.

"Generally, I'm a good guy but this diabetes gets me down, taking the insulin, especially. I'm feeling better, my head's clearing. I'm Tom, by the way. Pass me those tortillas and that marmalade."

I did and he wolfed the food down.

"Where are you from, Tom?"

"I live in Florida, was an airline pilot. I had to take early retirement because of the diabetes. Just got married again a few months ago and meant for her to come with me. She keeps me on the straight and narrow, looks after my meals and my insulin, too. She's a doctor, an internist in Miami, smart and good-looking. There was an emergency case just before we left. She couldn't get away. You wouldn't know about those things, would you?" he asked with a smile.

"On your next fishing trip, she'd better come," I said. "Don't leave home without her!"

He laughed heartily.

"The launch is here. I'll take your suitcase. The guide can bring your tackle box. We'd better ride to San Jose together. Just in case."

Mad Honey

The pedigree of Honey
Does not concern the Bee—
A Clover, anytime to him
Is aristocracy
        -*Emily Dickinson*

Can you imagine the pouched ants of Mexico gorged on honey, their thin walled bellies resembling grapes? Many types of honey may be produced by bees, wasps, or ants and influenced by the nectar of many different plants. Honey is man's original sweetener. Honey possesses other less well-known uses. In ancient Egypt, honey was an embalming fluid as well as a preservative of fruits and seeds. Bird's eggs were poached in honey and traveled great distances.

An intoxicant through the ages, honey seduces the tongue, eye and nose. No wonder it is the chief ingredient in drinks both medicinal and celebratory. Mead has been made for centuries. The ancient Romans made a type of mead called *mulsum* which was honey, water and wine boiled together. In ancient Greek mythology, honey and milk were given to the gods as libation for the dead. In Chaucer's time, wine was mixed with honey and spices and strained. In some cases ale would be substituted for wine. In New Zealand, I purchased a delicious mead made of wine and a type of rosemary virgin honey. Virgin honey, the most popular, is obtained from bees that have never swarmed or from honey that flows spontaneously from the honeycomb. The enchanting aroma of Maltese honey emanates from the orange blossom nectar. Exotic Narbonne honey is obtained from rosemary flowers and is delicious.

Throughout time, honey has been used in ceremonies. Hindus place a little honey in the mouth of the newborn male infants in a ritual of purification. Curd, honey, and clarified butter are offered to guests at traditional Indian weddings. Arab feasts are noted for the abundance of butter, honey with bread. In Madagascar, honey and water are sprinkled on male children as a blessing prior to circumcision. Indigenous people of Peru offered honey in their sun temples.

Although this divine substance is much lauded, it possesses a darker side. Mad honey, obtained from the nectar of certain plants, usually rhododendrons, appears in written records twenty four hundred years ago. Greek historian Xenophon in his Anabasis described in 401 BC, an expedition of Cyprus, King of Persia, to Trabazon, Turkey.

"All of the soldiers that ate of the honey combs lost their senses, vomited and were affected with purging, and none of them was able to stand upright; such as had eaten much more were like mad men and some like persons on the point of death."[1] Greek historian Strabo, born in 63 BC, chronicles the destruction of "three squadrons of Pompeii's troops who were given mad honey by local tribesmen and then slain under its influence."[2] In AD 23, Pliny the elder, a Roman biologist, philosopher and soldier, described "a noxious liver-coloured honey" found in Persia and Gaetalia (an ancient district in Northern Africa).[3]

In more recent time, descriptions of mad honey abound, though often in obscure journals. In 1825, French botanist August de Saint Helaire described a poisonous red honey stored by a species of Brazilian wasp. In 1849, Moffat, a missionary, reported mad honey in South Africa. The bees had obtained nectar from a euphorbia plant. The milky juice from this family of succulents and cacti plants was used by Ethiopian warriors as an arrow poison and the nectar was reported to "cause even the bees a fatal kind of vertigo."[4] Sir Joseph Hooker, MD, a British botanist and traveler, reported poisoning by honey obtained from wild bees of East Nepal in his Himalayan Journal of 1855. Hooker discovered that these bees obtained the nectar from rhododendron flowers. In the October 1861 Madras Quarterly Journal of Medical Science, Dr. G. Bidie reported the symptoms of prostration in patients who had ingested small amounts of honey from the Coorg Jungle in India. The symptoms described included, headaches, nausea and thirst.[5]

The toxins in mad honey are called rhodotoxins or grayan-toxins. In North America, these toxins have been isolated in nectar and honey from azaleas and rhododendrons from California to coastal British Columbia and from the mountain and sheep laurel of Appalachia. The toxins in these particular types of mad honey are poisonous in small amounts. Two tablespoons can cause slowing of the pulse, heart block and depressed breathing.

The poison varies with the species of azalea or rhododendron. Along the west coast of America, the western azalea, the California rosebay and the white rhododendron have been found to be toxic. In eastern America, the intoxication may be due to nectar obtained from the calico bush or mountain laurel. Reports of poisoning have occurred from the Smoky Mountains north to eastern Canada.

Appalachian mountain people know of honey's potential deadly side effects. In the Smokies, rural people collecting wild honey will feed it to their hounds first. If the dogs remain healthy, then they consume what has been collected.

Religiously, wild honey has been favored. In the Koran in the chapter named "The Bee" is written: "there proceedeth from the bees bellies a liquor of various colours, wherein is a medicine for men." Palestine was known as the "land flowing with milk and honey."[6]

John the Baptist was thought to have eaten wild honey, the nectar gathered by bees from the date palm. In Sanskrit, the ancient Hindus termed "*madhu-kulya* a stream of honey or an overabundance of good thing."7

In contemporary times, unwitting consumers of mad honey have reported weakness, numbness around the mouth, numbness of the extremities, nausea and vomiting. The slow heart rate can be treated with the drug atropine, while continuing heart block has been treated with temporary artificial pacemakers. With modern medical practices, the effects of mad honey are rarely fatal, the toxicity of mad honey being known to Poison Control Centres.

In commercial apiaries, rhodotoxin from mad honey may be diluted with good honey and the toxic effects are lessened. Beware of mad honey imported for its exotic natural taste.

1 Rhododendrons, Mountain Laurel and Mad Honey by Kenneth Lampe, PhD., J.A Medical Association, April 1, 1988, Vol. 259, No. 13.
2 Encyclopedia Brittanica, 11th ed. Vol.13. 1910-11. pg. 653-654.
3 Ibid
4 Ibid
5 Ibid
6 Ibid
7 Ibid

Tubed

I was to be tubed. Thursday morning was my appointment for an MRI. Over the past week, while setting up my MRI by phone, the receptionist asked me repeatedly if I was claustrophobic. I'd replied that I wasn't. Or was I?

I arrived for my MRI. I was feeling a bit guilty and anxious about the examination. Guilty because I'd paid up front and jumped the queue. Was I really claustrophobic and in denial? Just then my daughter caught my eye and said, "Dad, I should have given you a valium."

Could I will my mind tranquil and would it continue to be serene during my sojourn in the tube? You see I'd read about the MRI tube and its isolation. My defensive operations would be at work. Would symbolisation, displacement, and avoidance kick in before or after the examination? The examination tube was too narrow to admit a "phobic companion." I'd given my credit card and made my bed, and now, by God, I'd have to lie in it. Alone.

My name was called; the time was up. My watch, rings and hearing aids were taken away.

I stripped and put on the hospital gown. It was open from behind, I couldn't back out! Now I was naked, deaf —and at their mercy.

With some difficulty, I climbed onto a narrow stretcher that led to a very complicated looking tube. An attendant placed a harness over my head and neck to stop any movement. Pillows were put under my neck, because of my arthritis, that thrust my head forward. My upper torso is shaped like a grizzly bear, my marked kyphosis like a buffalo hump. Now I was a caged animal. Would the pillows act as cushions?

Before the technician tried to get me into the tube he gave me ear plugs. I couldn't hear the tech's instruction but with many hand signals I realized I wasn't to swallow and was to put the ears plugs in.

Finally, he pushed into the tube—smooth as silk. The tip of my nose touched a thin green line that traversed the top of the tube. What if I had to sneeze? A call bell was thrust into my sweaty hand.

"Ring if things go awry," called the technician breezily. At least that what I thought he said.

This anxiety won't do, I thought to myself. I'll be here for twenty-five minutes, I need to make the most of it or at least muddle through. With my eyes closed, my thoughts moved to more pleasant peaceful things as I concentrated on not swallowing. Occasionally my eyes opened and crossed as they watched the green line that seemed attached to my nose.

The machine started up. The electromagnets began to hum as the number of revolutions increased, whirling around me. The magnets were encased in frozen liquid nitrogen, but I didn't feel cool. In my imagination I was a torpedo in a tube ready to be fired. "Settle down," I whispered, "you're only getting your picture taken."

Finally the examination was over and I was ready to be wheeled out. By then the pillows that were under my neck had slipped under my head; my nose was pressed solidly against the green line. I was OK going in, but coming out was a different matter. My nose was being pushed up into a nasal salute. I was stuck.

"Don't worry," a melodic Caribbean voice said.

"Yeah, 'be happy,'" I thought. Hands reached in from the other end of the tube and removed the pillows and the harness. There was crunching in my neck, then my nose was free. The assistant rolled me out of the tube and I slowly got off the stretcher.

When I tried to put my hearing aids in, they wouldn't fit. I'd forgotten to take out my ear plugs. Finally I got them in and on the way out heard, "You were great. You'll receive your MRI proofs in the mail. Have a wonderful day."

Snooper

When I purchased my new Senso hearing aids, they opened up a new world to me. I leapt into a new digital age of eavesdropping. The acoustic abilities made me into a mole. Perhaps, I thought, I could work as an uncover agent. Would CSIS, the FBI or the KGB hire a deaf old man as a snooper, I wondered.

The new aids are comparable to a Pentium computer. The processor samples "sound signals a million times every second," according to the brochure. It adjusts sound automatically and reproduces signals into mellifluous voices. I believe Senso does what it says—"suppresses noise and enhances speech."

This sophisticated device that fits into both ear canals is a BTE (Behind the Ear) model. These aids are a marvel. When I drive across the floating bridge to Kelowna every day or when I use them in an aircraft, my information highway becomes a freeway.

At these times while sitting with the aids turned on I'm surrounded by metal. The sound waves from cell phones or from the cockpit of airplanes are transferred to my hearing aids by "the electromagnetic conduction effect of the metal superstructures," so my audiologist says. When traffic is delayed on the bridge or on the runway, drivers with cell phones and air crew begin talking. And I become a reluctant spy.

Once a week or so, if the conditions are optimal on the bridge, I get snatches of conversation from the cell phones. I learn about business deals, the kids at home or school, marital spats. Once I even heard about a sexual tryst slated for the afternoon. Unluckily, I reached the end of the bridge before I got all the titillating details.

The most startling conversation I heard was when I was waiting on a Houston runway. It was between the pilot, flight engineer and flight attendant in the cockpit. The conversation started like this:

"When are you going to get that rudder fixed, its been malfunctioning for over a month. You call yourself a flight engineer but nothing gets fixed around here. We're going to have a serious problem if you don't get off your butt."

"Yeah, yeah, you pilots are always complaining. Sitting in your air-conditioned cockpit while I'm sweating it out on the tarmac. The rudder will hold up for this flight. When you get back, we'll take this aircraft out of service. Better fill in another report."

The cockpit door opened and the flight engineer stormed out. A new conversation began between the pilot and a woman. The plane's doors closed and we were wheeled out into the runway for takeoff before I could pick up....

"Hi, boys. That was quite a party last night at the hotel. I hate the lay-over here, will be glad to get to Belize City. I love the beaches, even got a new bikini. You boys are going to love it. Hope your ol' headache gets well."

Then the gorgeous flight attendant came through the cockpit door and started to prepare hot breakfasts. When she brought me the breakfast tray, I said, "that was some party you and the crew had last night at the hotel. You must have great recuperative powers. Thanks for the breakfast."

She turned a deep red under her tan and left quickly. I caught her eye a few times, she blushed but didn't come to take my tray away. On deplaning I didn't even get a "have a good day."

Three weeks later on the return flight to Houston from Belize City, we boarded the same Boeing 737. I had an opportunity to ask the co-pilot if the rudder had been fixed and was in good working order.

The co-captain gave me a quizzical look and said "yes it has been fixed but how did you know about it?"

It was then that I fumbled with my hearing aids and asked "what was that you said?" He looked at me, then high-tailed it for the apparent safety of his cockpit.

The Healing Eye of Horus

The healing eye of Horus represented both health and happiness to ancient Egyptians. In the mythological story, Horus, a youthful Egyptian sun god, wished to avenge the death of his father, Osiris. Osiris was killed by the god Set (or Seth). Isis was the wife of Osiris and was known as the patron goddess of healing, but she supported Horus in his desire to kill Set. Although she advocated Set's death, she was generally benevolent. Her temples of healing were hospitals staffed by women. The ill and maimed flocked to the shrines of Isis, where they hoped to be made well.

Horus and Set battled. In the heat of battle, Set plucked out the eye of Horus with his thumb. A goddess picked up the eye and reinserted it into Horus' empty socket. Mythologists say that Horus' sight was restored and Set was mutilated but not killed. Horus has since been portrayed as having the head of a falcon, with unsurpassed raptor's sight and the body of a man. The shape of Horus' eye is a modified picture of the eye of a peregrine falcon.

To this day, the healing eye of Horus, known as the *Udjat* eye, can be seen on the back of the US one dollar bill, at the top of the pyramid. The eye is capped by the apex of the pyramid and surrounded by rays of the sun.

If you are interested in your own health and happiness, you see a medical practitioner. On his or her prescription pad you will see a stylized symbol. The healing eye of Horus has been modified to the following:

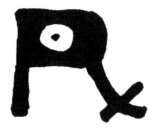

While the healing eye takes care of health and happiness, the *crux ansata* or *ankha* represents life and immortality. It was thought that the following shape symbolized the vagina, the vertical rod the penis.

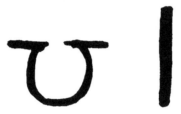

These were combined as the *crux ansata.*

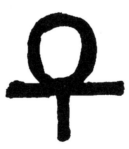

The symbol was the representation of immortal life and is now the universal symbol for the female gender and for Venus.

(Some of these stories have appeared in the *Canadian Journal of Rural Medicine, The Medical Post, AlbertaViews, Family Practice and the Harvard Medical Alumini Bulletin.*)